A Definitive Guide to Behavioural Safety

This book makes the case that far too much work undertaken under the banner of 'behavioural safety' is overly person-focused. 'If you can walk on hot coals, you can do anything – so be safe' needs to be dismissed out of hand, but also more advanced techniques based on coaching and empowerment fail to reflect the fact that, as 'Just Culture' models show, the great majority of causes of unsafe behaviour are environmental. Our methodologies mustn't focus on the person with an open mind that there may be an underlying root cause; they must start from the statistically proven assumption that there is an underlying cause. This shift in mindset has a profound impact on the type of methodologies we must lead with, how they are used, how they are perceived, and last but certainly not least, their efficacy.

A Definitive Guide to Behavioural Safety is a one-stop guide to all of the core theories and principles that underpin behaviour-based safety. All front-line behaviours that lead to incidents and injury are covered by the term behavioural safety, and getting to grips with the behaviours that might lead people to engage in unsafe or risky behaviour is crucial to prevention. In this book, internationally acclaimed behavioural safety expert Tim Marsh leads the reader through the three main strands:

- The awareness approach.
- The walk-and-talk approach.
- The Six Sigma safety or the Deming-inspired 'full' approach.

Going through the very latest innovations in the field, the book covers the systemic approach to safety observation, measurement, intervention and analysis, but also incorporates emotional intelligence training aimed at enhancing supervisor–worker trust and communication more generally. *A Definitive Guide to Behavioural Safety* is a perfect guide for any professional, whether you're aiming to set up an ambitious and wide-ranging behavioural safety programme from scratch or you're looking to refresh or extend an existing approach.

Tim Marsh was one of the team leaders of the original UK research into behavioural safety in the early 1990s, and is a Chartered Psychologist and a Chartered Fellow of IOSH. He ran the open courses on Behavioural Safety and Safety Culture for IOSH for many years. He has worked with hundreds of companies around the world, including the BBC, the National Theatre and the European Space Agency, as well as the usual list of blue-chip organizations from manufacturing, utilities, food and drink, oil and gas, and pharmaceutics. He was awarded a President's Commendation by the Institute of Risk and Safety Management in 2008 and was selected as their first ever 'Specialist Fellow' in 2010. The author of several bestselling books, Tim has contributed dozens of articles to magazines such as the *Safety and Health Practitioner* and *Health and Safety at Work*, as well as international magazines such as *India Safe*. Tim has a reputation as an interactive and engaging communicator and as a keynote speaker at major safety events all around the world, including the inaugural Campbell Institute International Thought Leadership event in 2013. Tim was made an Honorary Professor at Plymouth University in 2015.

A Definitive Guide to Behavioural Safety

Tim Marsh

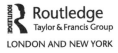
Routledge
Taylor & Francis Group

LONDON AND NEW YORK

First published 2017
by Routledge
2 Park Square, Milton Park, Abingdon, Oxon OX14 4RN

and by Routledge
711 Third Avenue, New York, NY 10017

Routledge is an imprint of the Taylor & Francis Group, an informa business

© 2017 Tim Marsh

British Library Cataloguing-in-Publication Data
A catalogue record for this book is available from the British Library

Library of Congress Cataloging-in-Publication Data
A catalog record for this book has been requested.

ISBN: 978-1-138-29051-8 (hbk)
ISBN: 978-1-138-64747-3 (pbk)
ISBN: 978-1-315-62678-9 (ebk)

Typeset in Bembo
by Swales & Willis Ltd, Exeter, Devon, UK

For my friends, the inspirational speakers Ian Whittingham (MBE) and Jason Anker (MBE), and the other workers around the world who didn't go home in the same condition in which they arrived.

Contents

Figures

Foreword

A little over a year ago, while sitting on a panel alongside Dr Tim Marsh, I was asked to help describe the elements of an ideal behaviour-based safety (BBS) programme. At the time, I remarked that some organizations currently treat BBS as if it were a long-forgotten Rubik's cube, gifted many holidays ago and left to gather dust after being solved once. As I listened to Tim and others far more insightful than I share their thoughts, it became clear to me just how true this glib statement is. Some of us may have 'solved' BBS in our organizations in the past (others may still be trying to get all the colours to line up) – but unfortunately for us, this particular Rubik's cube comes with an upgrade. The hands of time, culture and organizational change are constantly rearranging it the moment we lock it into place.

Tim writes in his preface – and throughout the course of this book proves – that behaviour-based safety is at a crossroads. The field has evolved tremendously over the years and become more nuanced – thinkers such as the author are to thank for that! We've come to understand the perils and pitfalls of BBS used poorly and the particular problems that arise when organizations apply its Skinner-based roots without deeper understanding, compassion, or evidence. Yet, even in organizations where BBS is well implemented and mature, a massive generational shift is pulling the rug out from under the tried-and-true approaches.

What's needed, then, is a guidebook that takes into account both the best practices surfaced from years of research and intervention, but also the necessity of tailoring one's approach. Years of exposure to excellent marketing have made all of us eager to find a silver bullet, but what we really need is a Swiss army knife – a set of tools that will help us in a myriad of situations, and the knowledge to fit each tool to its best purpose.

I believe that what you hold in your hands (or read on your screens) is just such a resource. Far from being a Rubik's cube, behaviour-based safety programmes continue to be a pillar of our work in the environmental, health, and safety profession. And much like those holiday gifts of our childhood, BBS has the capacity to create awe and wonderment when done right. Human beings are fascinating creatures, and when we turn our efforts to understanding ourselves, we uncover opportunities to do great things. Behaviour-based safety is among them.

I would caution you to use this book wisely, but the author has made it difficult to do anything but. Instead, I will urge you to not only implement what is set forth here, but capture and celebrate your successes along the way. BBS is a positive force for change, and is best when shared broadly and owned by everyone within an organization. I hope that one day I may see you on a panel such as the one I sat on with Tim – and hear how this book helped you to keep yourself and others safe.

John Dony
Director, Campbell Institute
Director, Environmental, Health, Safety & Sustainability
National Safety Council
Chicago, Illinois
9 September 2016

Preface

This book is an attempt to provoke a debate about behaviour-based safety (BBS), which I believe has reached a crossroads and requires a major shift in thinking.

Far too many approaches around the world either simply exhort workers to 'try harder' or use methodologies that attempt to coach people out of bad behaviours, or to change their values so that the same result is achieved.

With Just Culture analysis, as described and defined by James Reason and Sidney Dekker, showing that typically 90% of the cause of unsafe behaviour is organizational, such approaches will not produce the step change in safety thinking and practice that's needed.

If we are to maximize behaviour change, we must focus on holistic methodologies that analyze the causes of behaviour, as well as facilitate changes to the environments that foster it.

This is a weighty subject, and it helps that there's a huge amount of common agreement around the work of academics such as James Reason, Sidney Dekker and Andrew Hopkins, and academics and consultants such as Aubrey Daniels, Scott Geller and Dominic Cooper. There's a lot of excellent writing around key principles to build on, but I would like to take the debate further.

Critically, *there is no single definitive BBS approach*, and there never can be, as no one size will ever fit all. The best way forward is to select something that's broadly suitable to a relevant situation and then tailor it or design something bespoke to address it.

This book therefore follows the principles of a good job specification that helps accurately select the best candidate. With BBS, as with a job description, there are *essentials* and then merely *desirables*. There is a danger of confusing the two. Some insist that a desirable is an essential, while others ignore an essential or two completely.

Over the last 20 years, I have written dozens of articles and blogs, as well as several books and footage for YouTube, aiming to cover the full range of issues under the BBS banner, from the chief executive's office to shop-floor empowerment, plus all points in between.

Much of it has been deliberately provocative and designed to stimulate comment. It has left me bullish enough to put my hand up and say that I feel I'm as well placed as anyone to start the clarifying debate that we need.

Pedantic arguing among ourselves means that lives, limbs and eyes are lost. The most effective behavioural approaches focus on the environment before the individual. So let's stop using ominous and potentially threatening words such as 'behaviour' and talk instead about 'culture'.

Rather than lecturing people about their behaviours, we need to build a strong culture *from which safe behaviours flow naturally*.

If we do that effectively, then not only does genuine 'bad behaviour' stand out more; it will also be more legitimate to target it directly.

This book attempts to lay out a series of essentials and desirables for that debate.

Introduction

Behavioural safety: where are we now?

What is behaviour-based safety? How does it need to develop and how can it contribute to a new way of addressing the safety issues that exist in society, workplaces and our everyday environment?

BBS is a collective term for any safety improvement process or initiative that is primarily focused on front-line worker behaviour. The American E.S. Geller, who coined the term, has essentially defined it as 'focusing on what people do, analyzing why they do it, and then applying a research-supported intervention strategy to improve it'.

This book will argue that jumping over the cause to focus solely on the behaviour with person-focused methodologies is inefficient. Geller and others draw very heavily from the Skinner model of behaviour change, which encourages the use of praise to change behaviours. They have also incorporated good-quality coaching techniques to engender 'discovered' or intrinsic learning.

However, if 90% of the cause of unsafe behaviour is organizational, then we need to take a more holistic and integrated approach that draws on sociology. The Australian Andrew Hopkins has already done some effective work on this, popularizing the concept of the 'mindful' safety culture with books on the Texas City and Deepwater Horizon disasters.

We also need to change the terminology around BBS. Behavioural safety is too didactic and promotes negative responses.

Overview of approaches

I believe that behavioural safety should be grouped into five broad categories:

(1) The emotionally resonant 'awareness-raising' approach

This is a collective expression for personal testimony presentations, often from someone who has suffered a life-changing injury. Typically, they will discuss how, if they could have just five seconds back to make a different decision at a given time, they wouldn't have been blinded, paralysed or maimed.

The inference is that if you don't pause and make the right decision when in a similar situation, then *you* too could end up like them. Some of these arguments are extremely articulate, heartfelt and powerful, and will generate a major improvement in safety behaviour. However, their effect is usually extremely short-term. People are scared for a week or so before drifting back to their old behaviours.

While these 'be careful or you could end up hurt like me' approaches are face-valid and resonant, they are largely ineffective in the medium- to long-term.

(2) The STOP approach

Imagine a safety policy where management proactively tours sites looking for workers to talk to about safety, rather than just reactively pulling up workers as and when they see something wrong.

Originally developed by DuPont, there are 1,001 commercial and in-house variations of the so-called STOP approach around the world. They are behaviourally aware and driven through the line that demonstrates a genuine commitment to safety, as there is an investment of time and resources, but often they are also too top-down and far too full of blame. We could call this 'the don't approach'. In psychological terms, it represents an organization viewing safety not from an adult-to-adult perspective, but as a *critical* parent.

Transactional analysis theory argues that each individual interacts with another from one of three positions – parent, adult and child. The child is immature, the adult is rational, and the parent can be either paternal or authoritarian. Ideally, all interactions will be adult-to-adult or inevitably an unintended consequence will follow. For example, a paternal parent is a perfectly pleasant interaction, but means that the 'parent' is unlikely to be listening to the other person as an equal (they know best!). This will necessarily hinder any empowerment opportunity.

The STOP approach suggests that management can be either adult-to-adult or parent-to-child in approach. However, I believe that the emphasis should be not so much on what people are doing, but *how* they are doing it, and how it's perceived by the adults that they are doing it to.

STOP approaches at least demonstrate that an organization values safety and is committed to devoting time and resource to it, but they can be horrible, often counterproductive ways to approach the issue. I, probably like you, have responded badly to someone coming at me from the 'critical parent' perspective ever since I was about 10. STOP approaches can sometimes achieve excellent results, but there is also a price to pay from an empowerment perspective and, carried out badly, they can be worse than taking no action at all.

(3) A nurturing parent-style STOP approach

These methods contain an explicit element of objective learning as well as coaching. The SUSA approach used by John Ormond in the UK, for example, has nine clear steps encouraging supervisors to use *coaching* and *discovered learning* techniques as well as feedback.

Nurturing-style STOP approaches win awards and feel much more pleasant for a workforce, but do not lead to an apportioning of time and effort in line with what's actually happening on the shop floor and why. They will therefore normally not prove as effective as something squarely based on objective analysis.

Some learning isn't enough, but any BBS methodology or culture that doesn't have learning as its explicit cornerstone is flawed. Consider asking the question 'Why aren't you following the rules?' in two very different ways. An aggressive use of the query suggests that the listener is an idiot. A gentler application infers curiosity, not instruction. The difference totally transforms perceptions.

There was, for a while, a strand of BBS whose marketing suggested it was 'advanced behavioural safety'. Its exponents suggested that neurolinguistic programming techniques (NLPs) could be used to eradicate those lingering behavioural issues. However, the argument often used by trade unions that behavioural approaches should focus on the environment, rather than on individuals, is not addressed at all by a strategy that simply focuses on a person *really well*.

(4) 'Six Sigma' safety

W.E. Deming was an American engineer and statistician credited with inspiring the Japanese post-war industrial boom. He studied systems, their variation and how the human factor impacts on efficiency, and is considered the father of Total Quality Management and Continuous Improvement. Six Sigma is perhaps the best-known current variant of his systemic approaches, and was famously endorsed by business leaders including former General Electric chief executive Jack Welch.

Deming's approach involves analysis as well as workforce involvement and, commonly, measurement too. Applied to BSS, it adds goal-setting sessions and feedback charts to the methodologies that can be implemented.

Many of these approaches can boast decades of ongoing success. But can one really apply systems of proven excellence to behavioural safety when the whole essence of accidents is that they are not supposed to happen?

(5) A cultural or holistic approach

Based squarely on the Just Culture model, I believe this is the best behavioural safety approach. The Just Culture model works on the principle that the reason for an unsafe act is environmental, not personal, about 90% of the time. Therefore, logic dictates we should spend around 90% of our time and resources *analysing and improving the environment in which we want behaviour to be safe*, and just 10% looking at the individuals concerned.

This isn't a political or philosophical view; it's just cold logic. Once we accept that the first thing we need to do is to facilitate safe cultures and environments, we can get creative and can step into the world of behavioural economics. The nudge theory beloved of governments to encourage their citizens to adopt prescribed behaviours is an example of the use of such advanced influencing skills.

This loops back into techniques such as those on courses that, for a while, were offered under the banner of 'advanced behavioural safety'. These courses didn't simply use coaching to engender discovered learning and intrinsic motivation through standard techniques such as praising and questioning. They added NLP techniques such as mirroring, copying body language, including leaning forward or back and clasping or unclasping hands, to try to speed the development of a rapport.

Alternatively, an NLP exponent may use the same sort of terminology that the person you're trying to influence uses. So if you see a problem, they see a problem too. If you say 'It sounds good to me', they'll respond deliberately with 'I hear you'.

This is again entirely person-focused, and can actually backfire. If you genuinely listen to someone, then mirroring comes naturally. Mirroring clumsily comes over as a bit weird and is very off-putting!

In essence, the position that this book outlines is this:

> *Methodologies that treat all behaviours as an end in themselves are severely limited. Methodologies that also treat behaviours as cultural indicators don't go far enough. Behaviours should always be treated as primarily stemming from certain cultures, though some, once fully analysed and understood, may need to be directly targeted. This is not primarily for political reasons, but because it is more effective. It will change more behaviours for longer than other methods, maximizing the reductions that can be made in exposure to risks.*

Unsafe behaviour must be assumed to be caused by the culture, and therefore as an indicator of a weakness in that culture. Though the behaviour may not need to be addressed directly, especially if it presents a clear and present danger, we must primarily treat it as a sign that something is wrong with the organization, not the person.

Bad behaviour

'I want to talk to you about your *behaviour*' is almost never a good way to start a conversation for the person on the receiving end. It's simply almost impossible to construct a sentence with the words 'your behaviour' in it that doesn't sound ominous and put people on the back foot before we even get started. Using a term such as cultural safety or creating a safe culture would help reset and reframe the debate.

We all know something about the roots of behaviourism. It's about bells, Russian psychologists and salivating dogs. It's about pigeons in cages pecking buttons for food watched by men in white lab coats. It's about 'operant' and 'classic' conditioning. Classically conditioned responses such as salivating and flinching with fear, as studied by Pavlov, are instinctive, while, as Skinner has pointed out, operant responses, such as pigeons crossing a cage to peck at a panel when a light comes on, are behavioural.

Operant conditioning is used most in safety management, of course, but classical conditioning has uses there too. The worker who instinctively understands that the expression 'I want this safely but by Friday' means 'by Friday please (if you know what's good for you)'. He or she who responds accordingly is responding 'classically'. It's an unspoken and often largely subconscious reaction.

Language therefore has an important, if hard to control, role in effective behavioural safety approaches.

Using the right words, and thus the correct prompts, for desired reactions is enormously important, underpinning many essential elements of culture-change programmes. Yet, it also almost inevitably sounds like Orwellian mind control, and I suspect that the very mention of it instinctively triggers the rebel in us.

Similarly, we'd be advised to keep away from an 'investigation of an unsafe behaviour'. Who wants to be the subject of an '*investigation*'? The expression 'analysis of risk' is less likely to make someone defensive.

It follows that a genuinely comprehensive view of behavioural safety needs to be holistic, encompassing anything and everything that impacts on an individual's behaviour. 'Proactively building a positive, mindful safety culture' doesn't trip off the tongue like 'BBS', but something like 'Total Safety' broadly encompasses it. It's not just about the absence of harm; it's about the creation of barriers. These could be physical blocks on certain behaviours, as well as cleverly designed systems of operation that have the same effect. But it could also be simply about holding a handrail as a defence against gravity or a 'time out for safety' dynamic risk assessment as a defence against thoughtlessly pushing on when circumstances have changed.

Unsafe behaviour is merely a warning that things are going awry and could get worse. Todd Conklin, the author of *Pre-Accident Investigations*, uses the analogy of the warning strips at the side of the road that make the car judder if you lose attention and drift offline. Andrew Hopkins says that the key is to be mindful and to accept that there are *always* things going wrong. The trick is to go out and proactively find the red warning flags, not wait reactively for them to find you.

Conklin's thinking is essentially the 'new view' of Sidney Dekker, which is essentially summed up by the Elvis Presley quotation about the importance of 'walking a mile in a man's shoes before you judge them'. While Conklin exhorts investigators to reconstruct the roles of people contributing to accidents, Dekker exhorts us to move human assessments and actions back into the flow of events they helped cause to *understand why assessments and actions made sense to people at the time*. Dekker, in *The Field Guide to Understanding Human*

Error, says that when we look back with the benefit of hindsight bias, it's easy to say 'they zigged when they clearly should have zagged'. However, if we can reconstruct the situation at the time accurately and with suitable empathy, we can often see that both zigging and zagging looked similarly plausible to any reasonable person *at the moment in time*.

Reason suggests that safety barriers are like slices of Swiss cheese. The more holes there are up and down the chain of slices, the more likely holes are to line up and result in someone getting hurt. Consider this example. At the strategic end of a company, management agrees a work process that requires personal protective equipment rather than an integrated guarding system, which would be more efficient but also more expensive. In the middle section, the purchasing department then buys poor-quality gear that's uncomfortable to wear and supervisors seldom pick up on this. Soon, an individual who isn't wearing their glasses gets some swarf thrown up by a machine that blinds them.

This may sound simple, stressing as it does that safety isn't just an absence of bad events; it's the presence of defences. Reason's 'layers of defence' Swiss cheese model is a simple but powerful theory. It reflects the basic safety hierarchy, which starts with *designing out the risk* and progresses through *managing the risk*, ending with individual behaviour as the last line of defence. Einstein's relativity equation $E = MC^2$, meanwhile, is also simple but profound. It's the only one some of us can quote! I understand that it means energy is equal to mass multiplied by the speed of light, but this simple reasoning predicted the 'wobble in time' that was recently observed to widespread scientific excitement.

What I'm proposing is that, unless analysis proves otherwise, we need a mindset that treats unsafe behaviour as a helpful warning sign, not as a problem in itself.

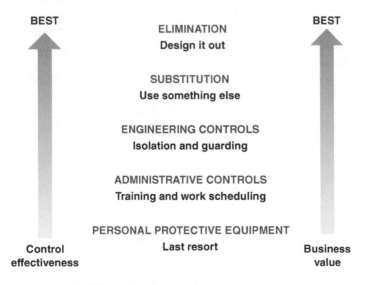

Figure I.1 The Hierarchy of Controls

We need to ask why a behaviour occurred with curiosity, not aggression, and to continue to dig until we find the behaviour's root cause. There will be a reason why people are risking their eyes by not wearing goggles. Are they aware that there is a genuine risk or is it simply a rule they consider to be over-kill? Is it actually overkill? If there is a risk and they are aware of it, are they continuing to not wear goggles because it is inconvenient or uncomfortable as they mist up and impair vision, or because they are difficult to get hold of? Could the task be redesigned so that the goggles aren't required?

Similarly, in *The Human Contribution*, Reason talks about an overstretched elastic band model, suggesting that in this imperfect world there will always be tension in a system, but that this is fine so long as things are in balance. Reason suggests that getting the balance right between safety and productivity means behaving in a way congruent with the statement that 'we want to be profitable and dynamic enough to keep ahead of competitors without hurting anyone'. The model suggests that when systems are set up, trained up and put in files, all is calm – the knot in the band is in the middle, in genuine balance. However, as life's realities bite, we can be pulled away from balance and drift into a situation where risk is too great.

Examples include facing competition from abroad, changes to raw material prices, or subcontractors that talk a great fight but then don't deliver. In essence, therefore, the strength of an organization's safety culture could

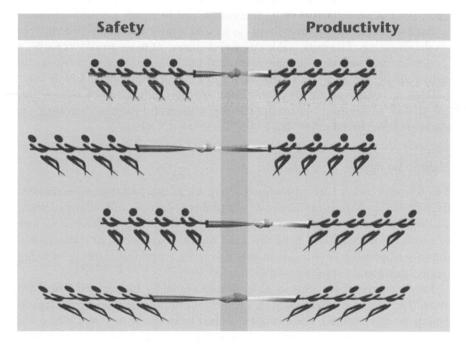

Figure I.2 The Knot in the Rubber Band (Source: adapted from Reason 2008)

be said to reflect the speed with which we spot that we have drifted and the speed and efficacy with which we are able to snap back into balance. Everything we do in safety contributes to this simple model. The quality of the systems and procedures we produce, audits, management walk-and-talk observations and behavioural safety systems, all feed into to this metric, which measures how quick we spot a problem and how quickly we're able then to respond.

We want to make a profit but we don't want to cause any harm in the process. Reason suggests that, because of complicating factors, such as bad weather, a change in raw material prices, subcontractors who talk a good fight but let us down, legislation changes, and the arrival of foreign competition from a developing country with cheaper labor, we will, from time to time, lose focus and have the knot in the elastic band drift away from balance towards unacceptable risk.

The factor that distinguishes the best organizations from the poor or the merely good is the speed with which they spot the drift and can snap back into balance. Too much unsafe behaviour constitutes drift. Objective analysis as to why it is occurring is, I'd argue, the most proactive and powerful tool in applying resources effectively so that we can snap back.

All this means that I'm arguing that now is the time to bury the term 'behavioural safety' forever. Not in terms of its methodologies and principles, of course, but with reference to the terminology. We need to dump the term because it carries too much baggage now, resulting in the positions of trade unions and other detractors being too entrenched to enable a sensible debate.

Asking people about their 'behaviour' also almost inevitably puts people on the defensive. The only viable suggested change of name to date is Geller's 'person-centred safety'. This, however, reflects his view that we address the individual people *really well* with quality coaching techniques, and doesn't address the central argument of this book that we should address the person *last*, if at all, in a holistic approach. The replacement I'd suggest, therefore, for the term 'behavioural safety' has to be 'Total Safety Culture'.

Holistic but flexible

The five approaches I have presented above are in order of their typical effectiveness and sophistication. However, flexibility is needed, and an organization will want to cherry-pick the most appropriate methodology for itself *at the time in question*. For example, I have few kind words to say about an authoritarian top-down approach, but this is in part driven by a personal loathing of being treated that way.

However, the classic situational leadership model by Hersey and Blanchard insists that, in certain circumstances, a top-down authoritarian leadership style is exactly what is required. For example, it's best to be direct with staff where the implications are important and/or where staff lack competence and experience.

Similarly, an old-fashioned emotional-awareness-raising session might be just the ticket to kick off a safety programme, as long as it's part of a holistic approach. It won't achieve anything in the medium- to long-term on its own, but it does allow for an explanation of what we are going to do and why we're going to do it. If the presentation starts with something upsetting or dramatic, we'll at least have people's full attention.

Finally, it may be that some form of all-singing, all-dancing gold standard approach might simply be beyond an organization at that time so that, for example, attempts to collect accurate data very soon descend into farce and chaos. This brings us to situational leadership, the concept that certain leadership styles work better than others in certain situations. If low-skilled workers exist in a high-hazard environment, for example, then a command-and-control style is appropriate.

Situational leadership is a bedrock of many management training courses, and old habits die hard. However, Daniel Pink has suggested that the world has become so complex that this is now almost never the case, and that a collaborative approach is nearly always required.

Defining cultural safety

There are thousands of definitions, flowing initially from the analysis of the Chernobyl disaster of 1986. One of the most common textbook definitions, from the advisory committee for the safety of nuclear installations (ACSNI 1993), is that:

> The safety culture of an organization is the product of individual and group values, attitudes, perceptions, competencies and patterns of behaviour that determine the commitment to, and the style and proficiency of an organization's health and safety management. Organizations with a positive safety culture are characterized by communications founded on mutual trust, by shared perceptions of the importance of safety and by confidence in the efficacy of preventive measures.

That's the starting point of a chapter in a 1,001-page book to set up where a good BBS approach fits in with my own model of culture, based on Ajzen's classic model of planned behaviour. It suggests three core elements on which a holistic approach to behavioural change can be anchored.

Systems

If training, inductions and systems have yet to reach diminishing returns, then working on them until they do will have a significant impact on the workforce's behaviour. It's not very cutting-edge or exciting, but it should be considered a fundamental part of a holistic approach to BBS.

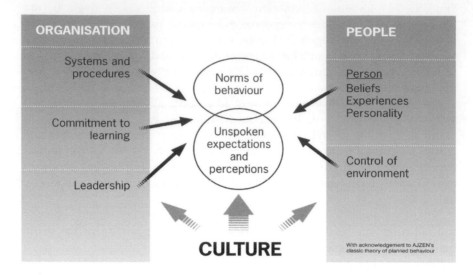

Figure I.3 Suggested Holistic Culture Model (with acknowledgment to Azjen's classic 'The theory of planned behaviour', 1991)

Leadership

Nearly every writer or researcher on the topic of leadership, coaching or empowerment agrees that 'transformational' leadership is preferable to 'transactional' leadership (meta-analysis of studies by Sharon Clarke and others confirms this view). Whenever it is practical, *usually* we want:

- the articulation of a clear message with integrity (otherwise, I won't know what you want or I won't believe you);
- using praise rather than criticism, since we know that is typically about 20 times as effective in changing behaviour;
- coaching rather than telling – to engender discovered or internalized learning;
- leading by example (because 'Do as I say, not as I do' stopped working when we were aged 6); and
- empowering (because, as Aubrey Daniels quips, if you're going to impose an idea on someone, it had better be three times better than theirs or they'll work twice as hard on their own).

It's not a controversial list, and any BBS approach seeking to utilize method-ologies around these principles alone will be a strong one. It will certainly be far better than something based on 'if you can do this, you can do anything, so be safe' fire-walking initiatives.

Learning

Though learning is the last of this trio, it is absolutely vital. As a species, we are our most progressive and enlightened when defensiveness is minimized and open-minded learning maximized. The Renaissance is an example of that. (There is, of course, the challenge to 'define progress', but I'm sticking with rapid increases in scientific rigor and social justice being good things). If it's good enough for the species, then it's good enough for a company BBS programme. To this end, I would argue that all BBS programmes have to have Reason, Dekker and Hopkins' concepts at their heart.

Some 'advanced BBS' programmes make no mention of these theories at all. Instead, they'll have NLP at their heart. But what all these *proactive* approaches stress is that we go out and systemically find what's going wrong, rather than waiting for issues to find us. As a consultant, I often use the Parker and Hudson model of safety culture as a benchmark. I'd estimate that 90% or more of the work we've done has been trying to get an organization that is broadly compliant but is struggling to overcome a 'diminishing returns' plateau to one that is broadly proactive. Reactive organizations, of course, tend to be preoccupied with more basic requirements.

I'll develop this reasoning in detail in the next section on why we take risks, but it's worth repeating here that objective study research suggests that 90% or so of the underlying cause of unsafe behaviour is environmental. Only 10% is down to individuals. Therefore, we need to spend 90% of our BBS efforts on analysis and facilitation.

It's not complicated

I'd like to suggest that the following simple model applies not just to BBS, but to all aspects of safety, health and the environment:

1 the risk;
2 the objective analysis of that risk; and
3 the commitment and tools to respond effectively to that risk.

This model should be thought of as an interlinked multiplier. For example, if we've designed out all risk, then we're fine no matter what we do next. If we do not understand the nature of that risk, then we'll be likely to shoot off on a tangent, no matter how committed we are or how hard we work. If we haven't the tools or commitment, then no matter how well we understand the risk, we're not going to be reducing it much. In short, we're only as strong as our weakest link, and clear thinking by the person on the ground is utterly key.

Here is a simple example of how this interlinks: If we create an entirely risk-free environment, then we lose the ability to identify and deal with risk when it arises. If there's no commitment to respond effectively to a risk, it is highly unlikely that we'll invest time in the proactive tools required to develop an objective understanding of it.

Some years ago, I was at a Singapore safety conference and met a man who said he'd been everywhere, done every job and had seen it all. I asked him which country was the least safe in his opinion, expecting a 'developing world' answer. Instead, he said 'New Zealand – they're very robust about safety there, they really are'.

It reminded me of a visit I made to New Zealand many years back, where I saw a sign by a small airfield advertising skydiving. I stopped and asked how much it was and how much training was required to go up. The instructor said, 'Well we'll kit you out and brief you thoroughly on the way up and off you go. So no time at all really'. I said, 'Bloody hell. That's a bit worrying, to be honest. When I looked into it in the UK, they insisted on a fair bit of training. What if I get it wrong, come over all panicky and forget what to do at the crucial moment?' The tough-looking Kiwi just looked at me and said with pity, 'I f***ing well wouldn't if I were you mate!'

As leading safety campaigner Ian Whittingham always stated, 'When it comes down to it, safety isn't complicated . . . so stay calm, think clearly and if you haven't the right equipment, stop.'

Section I

Identifying and addressing the problem

Section 1 covers some underpinning theories and principles. First, it covers the causes of human error and unsafe behaviour, and why knowing how to behave safely is merely 'base 1'. It also considers the power of Heinrich's principle, which is a universal truth applicable to all human endeavour, and not to be confused with the often dubious predictive ability of data associated with the triangle. Finally, it covers the vital importance of leadership.

1 Why people take risks at work

A nice clean categorization of behaviour used successfully around the world by numerous behavioural analysts, including BST, pioneers of commercial BBS, is:

- Non-enabled: It's not possible to do it safely.
- Difficult: It's possible, just not straightforward.
- Enabled: There's no reason why this can't be done safely.

For example:

- *I can't hold the handrail as there isn't one.*
- *I can hold the handrail but it's too close to the wall, semi-decorative, filthy, old, makes my hands dirty and sometimes causes splinters.*
- *There is a nice, clean, smooth handrail to hold.*

Unless we fluke it, anything we do to reduce unsafe behaviour has an upper limit set by the objectivity with which we understand the behaviour. That's just a law of nature. A BBS process that doesn't start with something as basic as this fails at the first hurdle, and will be just an initiative based on an intuition.

Just Culture: a framework for a systemic analysis

The Just Culture framework is more complex than the above three-option model, but still very user-friendly. Though not everyone uses it, many do, and it really helps an understanding of why things are happening as they are. It's almost as simple as 'First ask *why*', but it also allows a more nuanced understanding of causality.

The Just Culture framework was proposed first by James Reason and popularized by the books of Sidney Dekker and others. The book of that name by Dekker was famously the one that Captain Chesley Sullenberger of the Hudson River landing took on board to read when things were quiet during the flight. He didn't get much reading done that day.

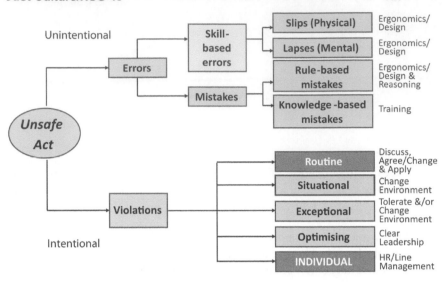

Figure 1.1 A variation on HSG 48 including some Just Culture

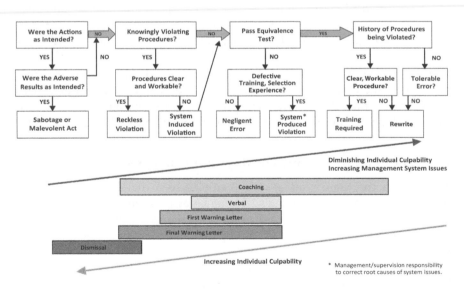

Figure 1.2 A simple example of a Culpability Decision Tree

Intentional or unintentional behaviour

Where an unsafe act has occurred, the first question is whether it was deliberate. If it was unintentional, then there was an *error*, and blame of any sort shouldn't be ascribed to the individual involved. Rather, we need to call in the ergonomists and trainers to address the issue.

Try this exercise as an example:

Stand up, stand on your left leg and rotate your right leg clockwise. Stop that. Now point at the ceiling and draw a figure of six in front of you with your right hand.

Now try the two tasks simultaneously. Harder? Or *impossible*?

Let's try to redesign the task. This time, rotate the right foot as before, but start the figure of six in the middle, not at the top. You should find this 'around and up' movement complementary to the clockwise foot movement, not contradictory, and easy to carry out faultlessly.

Of course, no one ever designed a task from a desk and failed to trial it with the workers who'd have to use it in practice. That would never happen! Nor would anyone put an employee in a situation where they need to be 'clockwise foot and top down six', then exclaim 'human error' when something goes wrong. Or would they?

Another example: at Three Mile Island, the control panels looked symmetrical and sexy but were difficult to use. The workers had tried to retrofit usability by using different beer cans (perhaps Coors cans for unimportant levers, Michelob for important ones – I'm not sure which, but you get the idea.) When the alarms went off, they couldn't be overridden so the employees, struggling to think straight in the noise, found themselves in an ergonomic nightmare.

Also consider the train crash at London's Paddington rail station that led to the second Cullen Inquiry. It happened when a driver drove through a red light. Initially, the operating company's view was 'driver error', the implication being that the driver wasn't paying enough attention. The investigation, however, uncovered that this signal was the second worst in the whole of the UK for being passed at danger (known as a SPAD). We'll never know for certain, since the driver was killed, but there's a very strong likelihood that he was paying full attention but simply couldn't see the signal because of the visual problem.

At Bhopal, workers failed to take heed of a gauge that was warning of a leak because it was frequently broken. It was only when the pressure gauge started to climb alarmingly quickly that they realized it wasn't broken at all, but had been accurately reporting worryingly low pressure. By then, it was too late.

Similarly, anyone who has tried to coach safety on the front line will have asked a variation of 'What should you be doing here?' and had the response 'Actually, I really don't know'. That's proof positive that a clear training need has been left unaddressed.

Distinguishing individual and organizational causes

Reason gives an excellent simple example of his categorization. He asks us to imagine an aviation worker checking rivets on a plane. In the first instance, the worker has the time to conduct the check, a torch to enable thorough investigation, and a gantry to support him as he does so. He undertakes the task diligently but misses a loose rivet. This, contends Reason, is out-and-out human error. We need to invent a machine that works better than the human eye. In a second case, the worker is lacking in either time or tools, and does the best he can under the circumstances. This is a conscious violation of the rules, but an organization-driven violation, and again the worker is blameless.

Moving to intentional *risk*

In a third situation that Reason describes, the worker has the time, the torch and the gantry, but chooses to undertake the task quickly, perhaps from the floor. This, he suggests, is a conscious individual violation. The worker is at fault and should suffer accordingly.

I once talked through this example to about 200 not at all shy and retiring safety representatives from the UK steel industry, and not one saw a problem with this reasoning. Actually, I think they *should* all have done so, since I want to contend that there are questions that need to be asked about that third worker.

Before doing that, we need to consider the can of worms that is untangling individual and organizationally determined violations. Dekker stresses that we must put ourselves in the shoes of the individual *before an incident occurs*. Otherwise, we are bound to apply some hindsight bias. This might be called '*Elvising it*' after the famous singer's reputed suggestion to 'walk a mile in a man's shoes before you judge them'.

This is where terminology needs to be precise. The classic definition of an accident is an 'unplanned event'. Violations are, by definition, *planned*, however.

The first is the 'situational' violation. This is where the task is set up so that something has to give, as there aren't time or resources to do everything. Forklift truck driving is a good example. During a test, a driver will stop and apply the handbrake before smoothly raising the forks, but has any reader ever seen a driver do that in anger? And if they did, what time would they be leaving for home that night? Now, there is still a behavioural distinction to be made between the driver who commences a smooth lifting of the forks maybe a pallet width or two out, thus putting the onus almost entirely on someone running through, and the idiot who drives around with their forks head-high at all times. Nevertheless, no one repeats the behaviours they displayed on the test.

Here's something you may have experienced yourself: You've driving to the airport looking forward to a well-deserved holiday with the family when on the radio you hear an announcement about a union work-to-rule that day.

Do you think 'Good, they'll be extra efficient and safe' or 'Damn, we'll be queuing for weeks?' And when you are strapped in safely for take-off, do you wonder which safety rules they choose not to follow on a *normal* day? Work-to-rule can be a devastating union tactic, but only because so many situational violations exist.

That's even without touching on the vagaries of subcontractors, peripatetic workers and piecework. The expression 'can of worms' could have been invented for the violations that these so often throw up.

Tell me what you want, what you really, **really** want? *(optimizing violations)*

Bizarrely, Reason doesn't cite the Spice Girls when defining what he means by an optimizing violation, but in essence it means stating 'I acted that way because on balance I felt that's what you *really* wanted me to do'. An optimizing violation is where the individual feels that, overall, all things considered, they are putting the needs of the organization first. It really is a manifestation of 'tell me what you want, what you really, really want'. In what is *clearly* (!) something of an in-joke, Dekker also refers to the Spice Girls' song 'Wannabe' when describing hindsight bias. 'We look back, with the benefit of hindsight and point out they zigged when they should have zagged', he states. (With reference to the running joke in the satirical magazine *Private Eye* – 'I thought I told you to take this out, Ed' – it must be noted that the editor remains utterly appalled that a reference to a lyric like 'zigga zig ah' is in this book!)

At BP, chief executive Lord John Browne demanded that cost savings be made across the business to improve profitability and drive growth. For a while, the managers at the Texas City refinery were much in favour because they pushed back little and tried their best to accomplish what was asked of them.

Consider feedback about a week's work where everything trundled off on the back of a lorry on the Friday afternoon in good time but where a few corners were cut to achieve that, with all relevant workers knowing that corners had been cut. Nothing that's considered too serious occurs and no near misses result, but if the management feedback is to simply congratulate all on a good job done, we can be certain that the same corners will be cut again next week, with risk mounting up until somebody gets hurt.

Certainly, when we see unsafe behaviour in clusters it is often because a 'common cause' applies, and frequently it will be about productivity. I once worked with a utility company where a massive spike in accidents occurred to the mobile sales force. They had suddenly started falling over and breaking wrists and collarbones at an unprecedented level. Some months before this spike, they'd been issued with palmtop computers, which they of course updated as they walked from house to house. They shouldn't have been updating as they walked, according to the rules in which they'd been trained. But it was a challenging and time-poor job, made even more so by the introduction of new technology.

When things go wrong, a decent lawyer will typically seek to defend an individual on the basis of precedent and custom and practice. Such arguments can get complicated as they need to determine to what extent managers and supervisors accurately or inaccurately second-guessed what senior management really wanted and how they passed that on. Senior management will then point at published core values and operating mechanisms that are supposed to ensure genuine balance. So we often have a situation where workers, supervisors and senior management stand in a circle pointing at each other.

How 'what we really want' is communicated: the killer 'but' and other subtle signs

Any expert witness will have seen other witnesses struggle to convey the sentiment 'I know it's true, but I'm struggling to prove it'. It's worth recalling the truism that 85% of a communication is in the voice tone and body language, even if we get the right words in the right order.

Consider this situation. You're at a table in a nice bistro with your partner. He or she takes a deep breath and announces, 'You're a really nice person and I really like you, *but* . . .' Would they need to finish the sentence or would you know exactly where that evening is going?

This is because we know that anything before a 'but' in a sentence is so much flannel, and anything after consists of the meat of the communication. Crucially, most verbal conversations are unrecorded so that when a worker is told 'I want this doing safely, but by Friday', they know exactly what's expected of them, but possibly may not be able to say how they knew when asked afterwards. If it reaches a court, a manager will state, 'I said "safely". I very explicitly said "I want it doing safely", so I don't know what the problem is or even why I have to stand here defending myself'.

Here's another example. Imagine walking into a bar when on holiday with your family. You're hungry and it looks nice from the outside. How quickly would you be able to decide 'wrong bar' without anyone even looking at you, let alone saying anything hostile or threatening? I would guess you would do so almost instantly, because the culture is, effectively, in the air around you. Leaving quickly, but still desperate for sustenance, you try a rougher-looking bar a little further along. The residents of this place look tougher than those in the first bar. Without anyone saying anything or even looking at you, how long would it take you to work out that you would be fine there? Almost instantly again?

The point is that when we are paying attention, we are able to read people really well and tell what they're thinking. Being able to provide for our families or just keep a roof over our heads means that, at work, we're tuned in to the most subtle of cues. Malcolm Gladwell, author of *Blink*, sums up this example, stating, 'If you walk into a bar and feel instinctively uncomfortable, you're an idiot if you don't stand near the door whilst you try and work out why'. (In doing so, he really rather neatly summarizes the Nobel Prize-winning *Thinking, Fast and Slow* by Daniel Kahneman.)

The reason that this 'instinct is often right' principle is important is that if we say it but don't really mean it, *everyone knows*. Again, we are hot-wired to give people not what they say they want, but what we feel it is they really want. The statement 'I want safety' is always trumped by a reference to productivity, unless the absolute relationship that a manager wants between the two is spelt out definitively.

It has to be genuinely:

> *'I want productivity of course, but I genuinely don't want anyone to take risks to achieve it'.*

If this is said with the right voice tone and body language, it becomes the start of a discussion about the logistical difficulties of achieving both.

Other examples of a supervisor or manager unintentionally or just subtly communicating a certain risk tolerance would include:

- Asking at the start of a safety meeting, 'How long is this going to take?' It's better to ask, 'How long do you need?'
- Saying, 'OK, but just this once'. It won't be just that once.
- Offering: 'I'll do it myself, but don't ever let me catch you doing this' on a risky task that requires knowledge or experience. Doing so will protect your team from risk on the day, but may not be such a good example on future occurrences.
- Announcing, 'Safety first, of course' at the start of a meeting, but then treating it like an item to be got out of the way as quickly as possible so that the really important items can be addressed.
- A CEO announcing at the start of an annual safety day that 'Nothing is more important than the topics that will be addressed today', before slipping out of a side door quietly to crack on with those 'nothings', hoping that no one will notice and that it isn't crucial even if they did. They always notice, and it *is* crucial.

To sum this list up: imagine yourself meeting someone in a bar who wants to talk sport. There will probably be some sports that you're much more comfortable discussing than others. So, how do you convey what it is that you're most interested in?

Actually, we do this all the time in everything we say and do. Committed people will devote time and effort to a topic, and do so gladly, not grudgingly or half-heartedly. They will have *opinions* they feel strongly about and will have an abundance of facts at hand, and will readily make time to discuss the issue. They will want to listen to your views and will want to convince you of theirs.

We're all like the family dog to an extent. Dogs are so attuned to body language that they can tell you're thinking of taking them for a walk before you're even aware of it yourself. It may be that two minutes before you consciously think of going for a walk you have the habit of breathing deeply and glancing

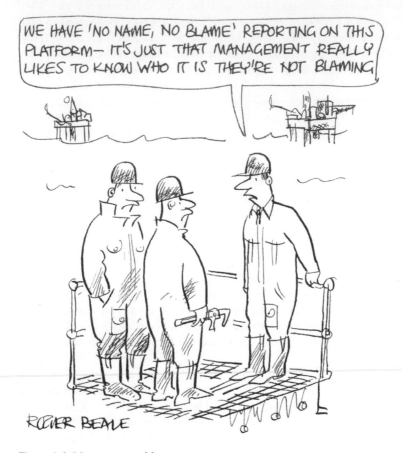

Figure 1.3 No name, no blame . . .

at the window. So, when you stand up and say, 'OK, let's walk, Winnie', she's standing in front of you, with her lead already in her mouth. Similarly, in a workplace, colleagues are often ahead of you and know what you're about to do better than you do yourself. That's why 360-degree feedback is so powerful, especially when it is about our livelihoods.

The practical implications of these truths

Once we start to objectively include such factors, analysis suggests around 90% of the reason for unsafe behaviours is *environmental*. Therefore, by definition, if an organization is to affect these behaviours cost-effectively, it needs to invest 90% of its resources on analysis, facilitation and culture building, and only 10% on the person involved. Management commitment and safety leadership is therefore crucial. That's not a political position; it's just cold logic.

Unfortunately, my experience is that many organizations instead run a 50:50 approach at best, with some behavioural analysis, but also a superb inspirational speaker – perhaps somebody blinded or paralysed in an industrial incident who can remind the workforce that it could happen to them.

These mistaken mindsets can be deep-rooted. I recall talking through this sort of material with an organization whose managing director responded, 'But my door is always open to anyone with a safety concern. I'd never send anyone away'. This man had a reputation for not always being approachable, so when I asked, 'Not even with your eyes?' everyone laughed. Luckily, he was good-natured and open to feedback, as well as quite intimidating. He asked if he did the 'I'm busy, so this had better be *really* important' body language thing a lot, and we had a constructive discussion about just how often people walked on, thinking 'It'll keep'.

The fundamental attribution error

The trouble is that we are all hot-wired to put too much emphasis on the person and not enough on the environment, especially when something has gone wrong. It's called the 'fundamental attribution error' (first studied by Lee Ross in 1967), and I'll return to it in the section on muddled management thinking. It'll kick in unless we make sure we make conscious efforts to stop it doing so. Otherwise, we'll see lots of the following behaviour – some of which you may recognize.

The rude Nike 'just pay attention' fallacy

Often, an organization that has worked really hard to design a safe workplace will look at the end-of-year figures and see that most of the accidents are frankly 'plain stupid slips and trips that could so easily be avoided, or indeed would certainly have been avoided, had the person involved been paying full attention'.

Often, management will also look at the volume of work pressures and fatigue issues, but conclude that there's nothing there to worry about. It's just the old adage of not looking where they are putting their feet. The solution seems obvious: an exhortation of the 'rude Nike' variety to pay attention to stepping squarely and to trip hazards:

*Just *&^&ing look where you're going! It isn't rocket science for heaven's sake!'*

Unfortunately, the human brain is a wondrous but easily tired organ, capable of concentrating for around 55 minutes an hour when rested, healthy and free from medication.

If you have an organization of 20,000 employees worldwide, that's an awful lot of unavoidable 'zombie' time mounting up every hour and every day. One way to tackle this is to exhort, 'Don't be a zombie. Pay full attention at all times'. But a better way is to say, 'If you see a trip or slip hazard in 50 minutes or so of alertness, stop and tidy it up so it's not there to catch you out 15 minutes from then when you come around the corner in zombie mode'.

Until we are all replaced by machines, the latter approach is simply much more effective.

The 'natural selection' fallacy

The 'Darwin Awards' are wonderful, detailing the 1,001 ingenious ways that people can do themselves in. It's a delight to come over all smug and chuckle to ourselves that being that stupid must have taken years of dedication and practice. On a more personal level, we hear that Uncle Ernie has succumbed to lung cancer at 65 and think that it was nigh on inevitable, with his 30 years of smoking 40 cigarettes a day. And at work we read about a worker crushed to death because he or she failed to follow a clear and simple procedure, and think how easy it would have been to avoid that outcome, adding the rejoinder, 'But if you play with matches . . .'.

It doesn't help that we are hard-wired to make the world 'fair' and balanced and to reassure ourselves it won't happen to us, by knee-jerk blaming of the victim. Hardly anyone is immune from this. We might say, 'That wouldn't happen to me, I don't go to football matches', or even, 'More fool them for following such a stupid sport'. But, leaving aside our worst instincts and taking only self-interest into account, we forget that the people in charge of safety at that event are the same people in charge of safety at the stadiums we do attend.

Admitting it could just as easily have been us isn't easy, and the reason the best inspirational speakers are so powerful is because they convince us that they are not unusual in any way, but, a stroke of bad luck aside, genuinely just like us. We need to constantly remind ourselves that nobody is stupid when everybody is stupid. At this point, we need to consider ABC analysis.

ABC (or temptation) analysis

ABC stands for antecedents, behaviours, consequences. Most compliance-oriented organizations think that if the antecedents (training, inductions and the availability of tools or personal protective equipment, PPE) are right, then the correct behaviour will surely follow. However, research shows that it is *consequences* that have the most impact on our behaviour, though you really need to talk about them proactively before something has gone wrong.

If we wait until *after* someone's been hurt, these issues will often sound like excuses. It's very difficult to talk about giving in to temptation through the prism of hindsight when blame is hard-wired into the human psyche.

Indeed, I wonder if trainers saying 'job done' and BBS experts replying 'barely started' is perhaps *the* key thing that behavioural safety has brought to the world of risk management. Certainly, anyone who doesn't follow up in the medium- to long-term can easily deceive themselves.

Walk out of my training course primed full of antecedents and jump in the back of a van with a bunch of experienced workers, and the consequences of any behavioural choices immediately start to kick in. The most obvious way is when one finds that the safe way is difficult, or perhaps that, although it isn't that difficult, nobody experienced actually does it. Hoping that someone young and inexperienced will not 'go native' almost instantly, regardless of how strong-minded they may be, is naïve in the extreme.

We need to consider here the nature of safety culture.

Safety culture

There are 1,001 definitions, but I think the best is 'the way we do things around here'. This refers to behaviour that's so unremarkable on a typical day that people literally do certain things and no one remarks. Training and induction efforts are essential, of course, but they are the very definition of 'necessary but not sufficient'. There's a tipping point at around 90% where it's almost impossible for a new start or subcontractor to not follow the rules when almost everyone else is.

We have an instinctive urge to follow the example of experienced people when we are uncertain. Imagine walking into a sex club for the first time or a garden party at the White House. Assuming that you have no experience of either, you'd maybe get a drink and find a corner from which you could watch what everyone else was doing so that you can orientate. People might say that if they were at Buckingham Palace, they would tell the waiters to take

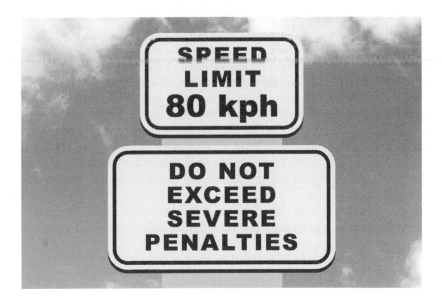

Figure 1.4 A clear rule with a clear warning

the champagne away and fetch them 'a proper pint of beer', but in reality very few would actually do so.

When collecting a car abroad, then joining the roads to be faced with a sign like the one below, we'd be very well prompted to drive at less than 80 kph. But what if, in practice, we find the inside lane is averaging 90 kph, the middle lane 100 kph and it's bedlam in the outside lane? The signage – call it the safety brief, the safe operating procedure or the induction, if you will – is crystal clear. However, at least half the people reading this would have used the outside lane within half an hour.

Culture is, by this definition, not what we say it is, but what it actually is. And it's hugely influential.

Case studies

The head of training of a large utility company, enthused by a leadership session he'd sat in on, once suggested a contract stipulating that, on the last day before they graduated, all apprentices had a half-day with our team to prime them.

We replied, *'If we tailor the course well, use our most high-impact and powerful messages and have you attend to close out the session, we can come up with exactly what you're thinking of and have a real impact on the day'.*

He then looked dismayed when we added, 'And it'll take some of them maybe *all week* before they go native'.

Let's apply ABC analysis to two cases that seem clear. The first example is a Glaswegian utility worker who climbed into a large hole to secure the bottom of a two-ton slab of metal while a colleague secured the top. The safe system of work was to secure it at the top and only then to climb down the ladder and secure it at the bottom. In this order, it removes an obvious and potentially fatal 'line of fire' hazard. In this case, they failed to follow that order and the slab slipped, and the man in the hole was crushed and killed.

My second example is a worker who was clipped and injured, though not seriously, by a forklift driver taking a shortcut on his second morning at work. Product was spilled and damaged, so there was cost and inconvenience to add to a deep bruise and small cut. There were 'Do not cross here' signs and clearly designated pathways, while the worker had attended a thorough induction, delivered by a manager and a safety representative who had helped write the training. He had even signed just the day before the incident to confirm that he understood the induction.

In the first case, an inquiry found 'human folly' as the sole cause. In the second, the worker, who was worried that he might be sacked, accepted a written warning about future conduct.

Before discussing these two incidents further, I'd like to talk a little about temptation analysis and *you*.

At conferences, I like to challenge audiences and prove an Aristotelian assertion that humour is merely 'common sense speeded up'. I ask delegates to stand up and then sit down when I stop talking if they have been guilty of any of the following:

- Driving at 50% above the speed limit (e.g. 100 kph in a 70 kph zone).
- Responding to an amber traffic light 30 yards ahead by accelerating rather than braking.
- Waiting until being behind the wheel the morning after a big night out before calculating the number of hours it will take to get below the drink-drive limit.
- Taking a drug given to them by a friend rather than a doctor.
- Smoking.
- Drinking their weekly allowance of alcohol in a single 24-hour session.
- Consuming sugar-soaked drinks, trans-fat-filled pastries and/or salt-drenched ready meals on a daily basis.
- Making a New Year's resolution to improve their health that they really, really mean but that they don't keep until the end of January.
- Having unprotected sex with a relative stranger whose sexual history they are uncertain of, though they look healthy and wholesome enough.
- Having had any sort of sex they shouldn't have (because if their partner finds out they'll be in trouble), but they are away at a conference or under the influence of alcohol, so all bets are off.

At the end of the list, 99% of the time *everyone* sits down. In a large audience, it's likely that several people will be innocent of all items but will sit down anyway to avoid the embarrassment of being seen as a 'goody two shoes'. However, the Aristotelian principle is proved when, having pointed this out, I then ask, 'As for the rest of you, is anyone tempted to shout "house?"' It always gets a good laugh, and there are always one or two people who seem proud to have scored so highly.

The point is that we are nearly all of us capable of behaving badly when temptation strikes, and the mechanism by which this works is explained by ABC analysis. The automatic assumption of many organizations is that if the antecedents are broadly correct and present, then the behaviour should surely follow.

But this ignores the huge influence of consequences that can follow quickly or be delayed, can be certain or uncertain, and can be positive or negative, because where there are soon, certain and positive consequences, there is *temptation*. Oscar Wilde joked that he could resist everything but temptation, while the British comedian Stephen Fry quips what he does with temptation is to yield to it straight away as it 'saves on the faffing about'.

Most of us are more in the middle in terms of temptation score, as most of us have our weak spots.

We all know that the list above contains the potential to cause us severe harm, including car accidents, HIV, diabetes, cancers and heart disease – issues that cause *tens of millions* of premature deaths worldwide every year. However, on a daily basis, we often give in to the temptation, assume all will be OK and enjoy ourselves, taking the shortcuts and consequent risks. This can be explained in part by evolution and physiology. Basically, 50,000 years ago, we were hard-wired to feast whenever we could.

ABC and safety, health and environmental management (SHE)

In the world of SHE, what this means is that if the safe or healthy way is slow, inconvenient or uncomfortable in any way, then we will be tempted to cut a corner and crack on. When we do this, risk mounts up and we roll the dice, fingers crossed. What's key is that 99 times out of 100, we get instant positive feedback. Not only do we get the benefits desired, such as time saved and discomfort avoided; we encounter no negative consequences. Accidents seldom happen, near misses can be shrugged off with a macho laugh in some organizations and health effects don't happen typically for decades.

Combine that with supervisors making no comment and we have a problem.

Just Culture, ABC analysis and the trade union argument

In recent years, many a trade union has written an article effectively calling BBS the work of the devil.

This is, in many ways, an entirely reasonable response to two factors. One is, from a union perspective, a perfectly accurate technical or instinctive grasp of the truth behind the analysis described above, even if they haven't heard of the Just Culture model or the physiological underpinning behind giving in to temptation. The second is that management either haven't heard of the model or haven't taken it fully on board, so cannot help but be drawn by the magnetic pull of expediency towards a person-focused magic bullet solution.

As a result, some managers tell workers that, since they walked on hot coals in a training exercise, they can do anything that they set their mind to, so they should simply go off and be safe. Others assure themselves that workers will be fine if they just follow all the rules they've been trained in, so there's nothing else that management needs to do.

The often heard truism that '90% of all accidents are caused by people and 10% by equipment failures' doesn't help. There are several variations, but all of them are a huge big red arrow pointing at 'so retrain and/or discipline the worker'.

It's better to think that 100% of all unsafe acts are caused by the organizational systems or culture until proven otherwise. We act on this assumption by asking 'Why?' curiously of things we've seen that are wrong, and querying 'Anything slow, uncomfortable or inconvenient?' about things we haven't seen or can't see.

Empowerment, workforce involvement and ABC analysis

Though it's jumping ahead to empowerment and the practicalities of other methodologies, I'd like to introduce a concept here that underpins much of this book with an improbable boast:

I could beat Roger Federer at tennis.

Yes I could, honestly, though I'd better explain why quickly. How good I ever was at tennis is irrelevant. The issue is not about me, but concerns why Federer himself is actually so good. It's because he's practised so hard and so long that his 'situation awareness' on a tennis court appears supernatural. He can read where a serve is going before the server hits the ball, not because he has better eyesight than us, or even better reflexes. (Giving a very specific example of body language reading, Andre Agassi has explained that he started to beat Boris Becker regularly once he realized that Becker had the habit of always pointing his tongue in the direction he intended to serve.) Actually, and surprisingly, they have been measured, and he does not.

Instead, it is because Federer can tell *instinctively* from the throw of the ball to the merest twist of a torso what an opponent is going to do, and instinctively respond appropriately. It's not a born skill; it's a situationally specific *learned* one.

In other words, people immersed in an environment see nuances, subtleties and interconnections to which other people are oblivious. It's like Eskimos who can reputedly distinguish 400 different types of snow. Federer has spent decades playing tennis, just as most workers have spent decades in their chosen fields. Aubrey Daniels is quoted as saying, 'I will only impose my idea on you if it's three times better than yours, as you'll work twice as hard on your own'. We hear this and see the sense in it with an implicit balance between education and seniority and local knowledge.

However, I want to challenge this. It is misleading because:

> No manager is *ever* going to come up with a local safety solution three times better than the workforce – unless they've bought a machine that designs out the risk entirely by putting everyone out of a job.

If we are to be world-class in our analysis of error, it has to be based on:

- not leaping to conclusions, but, as any well-trained incident investigation expert knows, first establishing as precisely as possible what actually happened;
- objectively asking why, as we are assuming there is a good reason; and, even more importantly,
- actively involving the people who understand the day-to-day practicalities and subtleties far better than we ever can, because it's really often all about nuance and subtlety.

As for my challenge match with Federer, I'd back myself to be OK at 'real tennis' – an old-fashioned version of the sport that Federer once tried as a gimmick for a magazine and was surprisingly hopeless at. Real tennis requires a very specific skill set, so if I had some notice and practiced really hard over a period of months, I reckon this would be sufficient to beat Federer. Similarly, Amarillo Slim, the world's most famous gambler, once beat the world table tennis champion *at table tennis* by insisting on the choice of bats. He turned up on the day with two frying pans, with which he'd been practicing hard.

If we are to have a world-class BBS process, it has to be based on an objective analysis of why behaviours are happening. This needs to be based on the active involvement of local experts working from within a Just Culture mindset and framework.

Individual personality

There's much controversy about the notion of the 'accident-prone' worker, especially when coming from a Just Culture perspective. Clearly, as a big fan of the Just Culture framework, I understand the reluctance to embrace the notion. However, my PhD is in personality theory, or specifically about the individual traits predicting suicidal behaviour in army recruits, make me feel well placed to comment.

Imagine you're on a plane with your children being flown by a pilot who is impetuous, aggressive, imaginative and creative, so easily distracted, low in conscientiousness, easily rattled and prone to overreaction.

Would you like to switch the pilot to someone the *opposite* of the person described? I expect that you might.

The good news is that Just Culture shows that these traits are not anywhere near as important as systems, leadership and culture, so there's less risk associated with an 'iffy' person in a strong culture than a 'safe' person in an 'iffy' culture. Sometimes, of course, we do indeed have an 'iffy' person in an 'iffy' culture, and Schneider's classic studies of the dynamics of 'attraction, selection, attrition' (ASA theory) between people and organizations show that these of course correlate. At this point, we have a problem, especially if they're in charge of something heavy, fast or likely to explode.

Of course, it's only a correlation. You could make the joke that NASA wouldn't employ an idiot. But then perhaps we could watch the film *Major Malfunction* and reconsider. There's some extremely suboptimal risk thinking clearly displayed there and systemically too. Then perhaps we could watch *The Last Flight of the Columbia*, where many of the same mistakes were made by the same organization, again with tragic consequences, proving that little was learned from the Challenger disaster. When we examine these situations closely, we find that suboptimal safety cultures were far more prevalent than the stakeholders would have hoped or assumed in the absence of conclusive proof otherwise. More than that, the NASA case study shows that even proof that any reasonable person would judge conclusive might be met by inertia and defensiveness.

Personal safety ethic (PSE)

Much has been written about the 'personal safety ethic', but a leader or worker can have one and still struggle to consistently act on it if the environment is wrong. I'm very sceptical about the notion that everyone can develop a personal safety ethic with the right education. First, we know from Just Culture that the environment is most important, and it's always potentially problematic to focus too much on the person. Second, some people are pretty hard-hearted and cynical.

With that in mind, consider this check-sheet.

1   Have you always had a personal safety ethic?
2   Have you developed one as the result of a (usually traumatic) first-hand experience?
3   Have you developed one through ingrained habit from being in a strong culture for a number of years?
4   Do you pretend to have one as you know which way your bread is buttered and can do it convincingly enough most days that few notice?
5   Do you pretend, usually unconvincingly, as and when you have to?

Another way of describing and/or measuring the success of a BBS or culture-change programme is to increase the number of 3s and decrease the number of 4s and 5s without having to go through the trauma of 2. Another metric is that we'll know we're getting it right when we increase the number of 1s that we attract to the organization.

Summary

We started this chapter with the plea that every BBS programme must at least have a simple triptych at its heart.

Is the task:

* impossible;
* difficult; or
* entirely possible?

In this chapter, I have tried to describe why carefully defining 'difficult' is so important.

In a blame-driven organization, the bar for 'difficult' will be set high and BBS methodologies will flow from that. In the worst case, this will manifest as knee-jerk blame and punishment, and in more enlightened ones individually focused 'try harder' or 'have a better attitude' methodologies, possibly backed up with inspirational speakers.

Both, however, will be ineffective, to a greater or lesser degree, and both will deliver unintended consequences harmful to the culture.

On the other hand, a Just Culture-based categorization will include cultural issues and cues to do with management and peers, and also human factors around temptation analysis. Systemically taking these factors into consideration will deliver a more accurate answer to 'difficult' and to the equivalence test of 'What would a typical person do on a typical day?'

The more accurately we address this in our thinking, the more effective the resultant methodologies will be and the lesser the risky behaviour.

BBS methodologies that don't have a Just Culture model at their heart will be improved by including one.

2 Safety training as ground zero

Mindsets that develop a holistic approach to safety are essential if training people how to behave safely is to become merely the first part of a thorough and effective behavioural safety approach.

One of the most important contributors to such mindsets is an appreciation of the simple principle that compliance is often discretionary. Culture is king, so the specific *interface* between *training* and *culture* is crucial if the message is to resonate and gain widespread adoption. Failing to follow this path is one of the reasons why many organizations have spent a fortune on BBS that looks excellent but gained little or nothing in return for the medium- to long-term.

This is a very difficult concept for organizations to grasp if they come from a command-and-control mindset. This way of thinking about safety officers in regard to their workforces effectively manifests itself as the claim that 'Not only have they been told what to do, we've given them the tools to do it and collected signatures to that effect. Our job, except to monitor and enforce compliance, is over'.

This could not be more incorrect. Studies have often proved that the average person judges unfairness much more harshly than illegality. It's the same with safety rules, which we may instinctively see as simply an attempt at a catch-all that will protect us from risk. Often, we'll see such disciplines as clumsy attempts that cannot only be inadequate for what they are trying to achieve, but can sometimes be completely counter-effective.

Rules are like many laws, seen as tablets of stone by those who write them and as a starting point for a negotiation to the rest of us. I once did some work with a European body, and was told over dinner that Scandinavian countries are difficult to work with at the legislative stage but much better once implementations began. Southern European countries, on the other hand, were easy to work with when writing legislation. The reason? The Scandinavians were far more worried about the detail as they would be the only ones striving to fully implement the new framework.

Maybe that was an unfair characterization, and perhaps things have changed since it was propagated, even if it did originally have resonance. However, on a recent European holiday, I was nearly run over by a helmet-less man on a scooter who was chatting on a mobile phone cupped between neck and shoulder and holding a steaming cup of coffee in one hand. I wasn't in Scandinavia.

Maslow's hierarchy of needs motivation model starts with basic physical and safety needs, moves through social and esteem needs, and ends with 'self-actualizing'. If you know of only one motivation model, it's probably this one. I'd argue, however, that the individual motivation model that best addresses safety issues is *Vroom's*. It perfectly explains what goes wrong at the training safety behaviour interface.

The model says that an individual's motivation to do something is a factor of three things and that these factors are a multiplication. This is important as it means that *a low score anywhere in the chain gives a low score overall, regardless of how strong some elements might be.*

This is really worth highlighting. It explains why a clear briefing about a genuine risk might achieve very little if a holistic approach isn't taken. Specifically, you'll see clearly that there's a need for *safety* and *human resources (HR)* to cooperate and coordinate.

The basic model is:

what and why × how to do it × perceived importance

What?

In organizations that have hit diminishing returns from systems and are turning to behavioural approaches, most safety briefings are very good on what needs to be done. Some are not and, where roles, rules and responsibilities are unclear, confusing or contradictory, we're in trouble before we've even

Vroom/Marsh Model

Why
for example:
– Heinrich
– Just Culture

Basic/generic skills
for example:
– Assertion
– Ice Breaking
– Presentation Skills

 X X

What
for example:
– Analysis
– Communication

More advanced /specific skills
for example:
– Five Whys Analysis
– Coaching

Embedding the new behaviour
for example:
– Day to Day Feedback
– Formal Appraisal Items

Figure 2.1 Vroom/Marsh Model of Motivation

got started. Similarly, if a workforce knows what to do but not *how to do it*, or knows *what* and *how* but hasn't got the *tools* to deliver what is being asked of it, then the 'behavioural' response required is basic.

Why?

The concept of 'operational dexterity' is known in a variety of guises, including warfare, but basically means that a team or individual has enough knowledge or experience to adapt successfully in a dynamic environment when things don't go as expected. They are astute in their realization that a plan B is required and are able to come up with an appropriate one. To do this well, they need a clear understanding of the underpinning principles.

In behavioural safety, for example, it is always advisable to walk through the Heinrich principle before a briefing on key behaviours that need improving, especially if they seldom lead to injury or haven't led to an injury recently, and a complacent overconfidence has built up.

Heinrich's triangle, also known as the Bird triangle, was conceived in the early twentieth century, and is covered in full in the following chapter. There's been a lot of argument about its predictive validity, but the principle is sound, which is that the more unsafe behaviours there are, the increased likelihood there is of an unwanted serious outcome.

Applied to modern safety, the hard hat we always wear on-site that saves us from certain death when a scaffold clip is accidently kicked off is a clear and visible example of 'breaking the chain'. Other examples of breaking the chain would be the recently replaced toe-board that prevents the kicked scaffold clip from getting 'airborne' or a good housekeeping policy that means that the scaffolding platform has no loose items on it in the first place. We need to 'work' the principle at the behavioural level and let the pointy end of the triangle take care of itself. Often, we'll never know who we saved. If it's the hard hat, then we know all about it, but not if it's the clear housekeeping.

Similarly, I would always suggest that the principles underpinning Just Culture and a quick review of Reason's Swiss cheese model precede a course on 'Five Whys' analysis or another root cause analysis technique. Five Whys is perhaps the simplest and easiest to use of such techniques, and frequently proves to be the most useful. The technique is simply not to stop asking 'why' curiously until the question becomes pointless because a fundamental underlying issue has been identified. You can, of course, ask, 'Why do they want to save money?', but unless the answer shines light on a hitherto unknown cash-flow crisis, the reason will be self-evident. Usually, this 'Now I really understand' insight will take five steps, but it could take six, or just one. There may also be several answers. The rule is simple. If asking why curiously makes sense, then an unasked 'why' question is a learning opportunity missed. (We'll return to this concept in a little while.)

However, time is money, and money is often tight, so some organizations skip the 'why' or do it badly. This means that delegates won't have the background knowledge to adapt successfully if required. This means unsafe acts, and the more dynamic the environment, the more likely it is that this lack of operational dexterity might prove costly.

How?

I remember an operative staring at a very expensive suction-based lifting tool utterly flummoxed as to how to use it in a way that didn't double the time required to lift something. He therefore left it standing idly by most of the time while he lifted manually as he always had. This wasn't good; the boxes in question were far too heavy, and the risk assessment stated: 'Provide a tool or make it a two-person lift'. The positive side was that one lifting tool was promptly installed. The negative part is that it was never used. There will be hundreds and thousands of similar examples.

A more subtle variation on this theme would be where supervisors have been trained in an interpersonal methodology, such as the classic intervention to provide feedback, but feel they don't have the skills to do so without making a fool of themselves. Do they go back to the trainer or their manager to request additional training, or do they avoid the task whenever possible? That's a rhetorical question, of course, and this just a more specific version of blind eye syndrome.

Similarly, where someone is tasked to give an important safety brief but is maybe one of those people who find public speaking scarier than death (it's about 15% apparently), then that will be avoided or delegated if possible. If that's not possible, it's likely to be a low-impact mumbled affair or an overly complicated slide deck read out word for word by someone with their back to the audience.

This is a behavioural safety issue. If there is a safety topic that needs a presentation, then it's important. If it's important, then it needs to be done well, and, at the very least, the person tasked with delivering it should have been through a half-decent presentation skills training course. In addition, anything involving communication, interpersonal or analytical skills really needs role-play and interactive exercises.

Considered important

Contestants in the television game show *Who Wants to Be a Millionaire?* can bank money at certain stages before pushing on.

Vroom's model, however, highlights the fact that nothing can be banked at the end of a training course, except perhaps skills that an individual can take *elsewhere* – no matter how good the course is . . .

Consider the following well-researched, -designed and -delivered course:

The techniques required were illustrated clearly and the background context was explained so the 'why' was covered thoroughly. The course was long and interactive enough for the person to play around with the techniques in role play in the comfort of a classroom and feel that they would be reasonably comfortable using them in anger.

The course was excellent, interactive, informative and fun. Delegates were treated as adults and the role plays went well, with the trainer kicking off with the old Scott Geller joke that illustrates that training isn't briefing because it needs to be practical and hands-on. The joke asks parents to imagine that their teenage daughter comes home and says, 'We're doing sex education next week at school'. The following week, she reports: 'The sex education went well, so we're moving on to sex *training* next week'. The parental reaction to this illustrates that education is not training.

This course also featured an exercise where 'Bobby' had to pretend to be an irate corner-cutting contractor so that 'Jim' could practise his assertion techniques. The reaction of the participants captured perfectly how it really is out there. Great, get those 'happy sheets' collected in and collated. Job done.

Unfortunately, it's not so simple.

Why this is so is neatly summarized by an old colleague of mine who worked in safety on shipyards around the world for many years. He used to say, 'If the things we ask workers to do aren't considered career-enhancing in the smoke shack six months from now, then they won't be happening and we've probably wasted a lot of time and money'.

Although it breaks my heart as a provider of training to say so, 80% of the effectiveness of a training course is in the follow-up and embedding of the behaviours requested. This means systemic follow-up through formal and informal feedback, and ideally coaching support. Even then, it's not just doing it – it's about *how* it is done. Having safety as an item on a formal yearly appraisal is one thing, but if the manager conducting it skips through it rapidly and then returns to a thoughtful pace when the session returns to other matters, it sends completely the wrong message.

Experience suggests training courses have some that listen to nothing and some that listen keenly to all. The majority, it seems, are what might be called bluff-calling sceptics. They've seen it all before and leave the course thinking, 'It sounds good, but then so did that last initiative, so we'll see'. For them, what happens next is everything.

Here's a trick for following up the embedding process to see how genuine the commitment is to the safety principles that have just been learned on a course. Film an operations-driven appraisal that includes some HSE elements, but switch the sound off and watch the body language. Is there a definite change of tone when the safety items are raised with all concerned relaxing before refocusing on the important issues? To misquote George Orwell, in appraisals some issues can be more equal than others. As ever, it's not what we do, but the way that we do it.

The following graph illustrates this really well. It's data from an organization that had a quota for 'walk-and-talks' that was linked to the bonus system. Unfortunately, they didn't cross-reference the quality of the interactions with the quantity. Again, the Spice Girls are the reference: 'Tell me what you want, what you really, really want'.

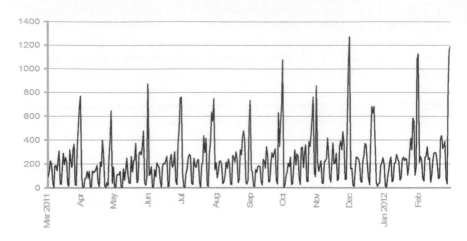

Figure 2.2 Daily Observations Graph

Personal safety ethic

An example of a virtuous circle moving an individual to developing a genuine personal safety ethic (PSE) would be via self-awareness and empathy. These can be enhanced by good-quality safety conversations through a formal or informal, but meaningful, walk-and-talk approach. Using 360-degree follow-ups to ensure that these are good-quality conversations where managers actively listen to feedback will help build a strong and supportive culture. Where this isn't going well naturally, or where an individual is merely going through the motions, one-to-one follow-up coaching can help.

Simply telling workers that they should all have a PSE, and, if they don't have one, they should get one, is a world away from a systemic, holistic, practical approach to building a culture of behavioural safety.

You cannot download a culture supportive of behavioural safety. You can't even attain one just through running the best safety training course on the planet. You have to *build* one. Constantly running excellent courses, perhaps interspersed with high-impact and heartfelt awareness-raising sessions, will keep safety at the forefront of people's minds and ensure that the safety performance doesn't degrade. But, without a systemic plan for medium- to long-term success, you'll plateau and find yourself with data reflecting the infamous safety wave.

Below is a classic safety wave and also the data from a couple of clients. Here's a prediction: half the people reading this book will be within an organization with data just like this. Actually, that's cheating a bit since, to an extent, it's a self-selecting of people who bought it as they are working on a BBS project *because* they have data like this. So let's say 75%.

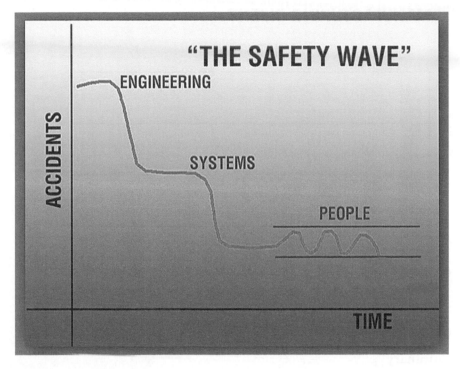

Figure 2.3 The Safety Wave

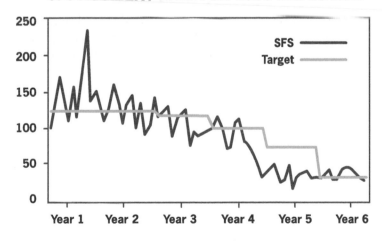

Figure 2.4 Client data showing a classic Safety Wave

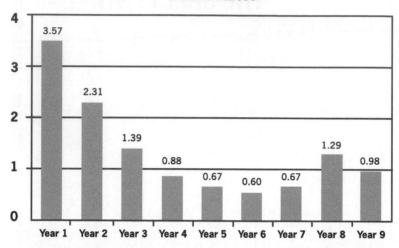

MANUFACTURING CLIENT

LTIFR Rates

Figure 2.5 Manufacturing client data showing a classic Safety Wave

Summary

Organizations build a strong safety culture person-by-person, day-by-day and behaviour-by-behaviour.

The key to continuous improvement isn't running an excellent safety course; it's the follow-up and embedding of the key behaviours requested on that course.

Start with an unsafe behaviour, then systemically walk back through the Vroom model to a training course, or even beyond that to a training needs analysis – if there is one. I have yet to find an organization that has not benefited from this approach.

3   The Heinrich principle

Based on the work of Herbert Heinrich, the eponymous 'Heinrich's triangle' says (classically) that for every serious incident, there will be 30 minor incidents or near misses and 300 unsafe behaviours. A follow-up study by Frank Bird found differing data, but a similar triangle-shaped relationship, leading some to refer to the Bird triangle, and a study by Fred Manuele systemically dissected the academic rigor of Heinrich's work and the difficulties of comparing 1930 work and data collection practices with the modern day.

It's an area that has taken a fair amount of criticism in recent years, with critics often quoting Manuele, but nearly always because the data doesn't seem to be entirely valid as a *predictive* tool. There's also the perception that with Heinrich focusing so strongly on day-to-day behaviour, he overemphasized the role of the individual and underplayed the role of management. (This puts me in the ironic position of arguing that we still haven't focused enough

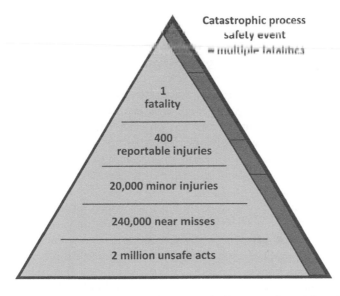

Figure 3.1 Extended Heinrich's Triangle (Source: adapted from Heinrich 1950 and HSE figures)

on the environment, as these critics suggest, while arguing in defence of the Heinrich principle.) Most infamously, this happened at Texas City, where a celebration of a substantial period of lost time injuries (LTIs) took place on the very morning of the explosion, with later investigations concluding that this was a 'disaster just waiting to happen'. This was proof positive that management weren't focusing on everything they should have been.

Such examples have led some process safety engineers to quip, 'I'm not going to stop my plant blowing up by getting everyone to hold the handrail'. The riposte is, 'Well, no, but you will stop people from falling down the stairs'. To take the UK North Sea as an example, more people have been killed in falls over the years than were killed in the Piper Alpha explosion.

Process and personnel safety *are* separate issues requiring separate controls and methodologies. However, this is only true to an extent, as there are also huge overlaps, especially when we consider the deeper root causes of something going wrong with either. The same manager who should challenge a rushed handover and request a quiet chat with a technician who said he would check the fluid levels later if he had time should also challenge poor housekeeping.

The fact that behavioural data is often a poor predictor of process events reflects two things. First, incidents caused by a lack of containment, such as leaks, explosions and fires, are by their nature statistically rare in most countries, and are usually caused, on any given day, by a *combination* of *several* unlikely events. Because of the nature of probability data, they are therefore very difficult to predict. Indeed, decades ago, they were often dismissed as just bad luck or acts of God. Second, it depends what you're measuring, and how well.

Holding the handrail is a prediction of lack of containment only insofar as it may reflect a weak culture. Fatigue issues, handover issues, maintenance and auditing issues, measured well, will indeed, on the other hand, predict the likelihood of an event. Insisting that engineers prove that something will happen, rather than accepting their professional judgement that the likelihood is too high, is something that Andrew Hopkins describes as a clear warning sign of a 'non-mindful' safety culture. This is exactly what happened with the Challenger space shuttle disaster, where engineers concerned O–rings might fail in cold temperatures had to admit the data was worrying rather than conclusive. (Having had to 'admit' that it wasn't conclusive, stressing that it was very worrying, cut no ice with management that had already dismissed their concerns.)

So a 'behavioural' predictor about this issue of degree of proof for process safety might be the question:

To what extent is your expertise as an engineer overruled for reasons of cost or political expediency? On a five-point scale, we'd want most of our engineers to respond 'never' or 'hardly ever' rather than 'often', wouldn't we? We just need a handful of questions such as this, with a stratified sample, asked in a format that encourages honest responding. We'd also prefer that, when our children grow up, they work in a factory that scored 3.8 rather than one that scored 1.8.

The core BBS approach of behavioural safety technology consultancy is the Behaviour-Based Accident Prevention Process (BAPP), which is essentially about identifying unsafe behaviour, measuring it, feeding it back to the workforce, and facilitating improvement. Even within this definition – about which they are very rigorous – the simple measure that I have described above fits under their BBS banner.

*Therefore, I stand by the claim that Heinrich's principle holds at all times and in every sphere of human life, and that the importance of 'working it' as an underpinning SHE principle cannot be overstated. The triangle is not always a predictive tool, though it can often be. However, it is **always** the description of a universal principle of profound importance.*

With the explosion of the Buncefield oil refinery in the UK in 2005, shift length and standard overtime hours meant that many workers were extremely fatigued. The worst approach is to blame tired workers for taking shortcuts or to berate them for 'failing to take suitable care where they're putting their feet'. Better than this, but still not ideal, we could and should say that many of the team are often tired and low in focus, so we need to make extra sure there's nothing to trip over or that we double-check the paperwork. Or we could take a holistic and rational approach and directly address the fatigue issue too. I have read of initiatives where obviously fatigued workers in the heat of the Middle East are sent off to have a quick snooze, because a 20-minute nap gives you three more hours of focus. Similarly, there was the initiative to give builders 'cheap bowls of porridge' during the construction programme for the London 2012 Olympics to prevent them travelling in at 5 a.m. on empty stomachs.

Both are excellent examples of behavioural safety as they directly address the cause of at-risk behaviour.

Its ubiquity and importance underpins the view that a behavioural approach is all things, but that all things can also be a behavioural approach. I was once asked to assess an in house BBS approach where soft skills training for management was the sole behavioural safety methodology. My response was to comment, 'Well, there are several other things I'd suggest you could do too – but basically it sounds good to me'.

The basis of excellence

Fascinating books such as Malcolm Gladwell's *Outliers* and Matthew Syed's *Bounce* provide plentiful case studies from the world of sport and commerce, showing that repeated hard graft is the *only* way to attain excellence. (Gladwell's book quotes the often-heard figure that though competence can be achieved quickly, it requires 10,000 hours to achieve mastery. He illustrates this with the story of Bill Gates, who was lucky enough to be one of the few people on the planet to have enough access to a mainframe computer to have got to his 10,000 hours as quickly as he did.)

It's not just about practice; it's about targeted, thought-through practice. For example, golfer Gary Player quipped that it was funny how he seemed to get luckier the harder he practiced. I always imagined him working on his bunker shots at dusk until his hands bled. Later, I found a (poor-quality) photo of him sweating buckets in a gym, decades before any other golfers worked out. I think it's an excellent metaphor. The Heinrich principle states that we get no guarantees either way, but that we can impact on how much luck we might need.

Even Mozart, the poster boy for the so-called 'born genius', was not really one. His father was a strict disciplinarian and one of the world's leading music teachers. Not practising hard really wasn't an option. Yes, he was composing while in short trousers, but most of it was rubbish, and he didn't write anything genuinely good until he was in his early twenties. Some musical experts even consider him to be a late developer. The Heinrich principle certainly applies to the world of health and well-being too. The Dalai Lama quips that his appearing to be happy all the time might have something to do with him practising hard at it every day for 60 years.

There are no exceptions. If you want excellence, you need to *graft* for it, so it's an eternal frustration of the safety professional to work for a board that say they want excellence, but in effect want safety excellence based on a gentle jog in the park once a week.

I find myself utterly frustrated by such individuals failing to get beyond the hope that there is surely a magic bullet for them somehow and somewhere. Take the delegate who approached Laszlo Polgar at a conference on learning and excellence.

In the 1970s, Polgar suggested that his ideas about learning and excellence should be adopted by the Hungarian government. They gave him short shrift, so he sought to prove his theories by having children to experiment on, advertising in a newspaper for a wife to provide the said children.

He found himself a wife who was supportive of his ideas, and in time three daughters arrived. He announced that he'd get them to excel at *chess* specifically, as scores and ranking points don't lie and the training was cost-free. He used a variety of innovative and empowering training techniques that had the daughters relishing every moment they practised, with the result that all three reached world-class standards. Judit Polgar is considered the strongest female player of all time.

After all this, a man approached him at a conference and stated, 'You must be the luckiest man alive. You have all these crackpot ideas about excellence, say they'll excel at chess specifically, and then only go and father the Polgar sisters'.

How do you convince a board that simply won't listen? You can discuss the notion of investment, not cost, the 'win-win' financials, use data and case studies, and utilize emotive messages that target the primal as well as the rational brain. But sometimes *you just can't convince them*. Whatever you say, you'll simply get defensive rationalizations, or worse, because you just can't convince someone who won't engage with an open mind.

Excellence always requires *targeted* effort.

Heinrich's principle and old-fashioned awareness-raising

It is worth considering a key point of the presentations of Ian Whittingham and Jason Anker, both excellent safety campaigners decorated with awards by Britain's Queen. Whittingham would ask, 'What happens when someone falls over?' and would get the answer, 'Usually nothing except embarrassment if someone sees you'. Taking this on, he'd point out that sometimes people fall awkwardly and break a wrist, a collarbone or even their neck, while sometimes they hit their head and die. Actor Liam Neeson's wife, Natasha Richardson, died after falling on a ski slope. She wasn't hurtling along, but barely moving on a nursery slope while learning to ski.

Whittingham's point was that once people slip, they've lost control, and what happens next is largely a roll of the dice. The trick, he points out, is to not slip and lose control in the first place. More slips mean more broken bones, more paralysis and more deaths.

Anker, meanwhile, observes that analysis of accidents with the benefit of hindsight shows they could almost certainly be prevented if we gained back a key five-second period to make a different decision or not undertake a certain risky behaviour, such as leaning from a ladder or stepping blindly onto something potentially fragile.

Here is a simple exercise based on a chapter in Bill Bryson's excellent travel book *Notes from a Big Country* to illustrate these points. Bryson muses amusingly on the sort of people having some of the accidents described in the files he considers. Natural selection in action is his basic position, and it's very easy to laugh along, but, nearly always, we're wrong to do so.

The categories he mentions, in alphabetical order, are:

- axes, hatchets and chainsaws;
- ceilings and walls;
- chairs and sofas;
- clothing;
- grooming devices;
- pens, pencils and desk accessories;
- scissors; and
- stairs and ramps.

One of these categories accounts for millions of accidents in US workplaces and homes every year, while three of them each describe mishaps in the hundreds of thousands, and five depict incidents afflicting tens of thousands. See if you can guess which is which.

Many people pick the dangerous categories, while others think about the risk assessment factor frequency and find themselves drawn to the everyday items. The actual answers are 'stairs and ramps' ahead by a country mile at 2 million, followed by 'ceilings and walls', 'chairs and sofas' and 'clothing', which are in the hundreds of thousands. (With reference to the Heinrich principle, it's worth pointing out that around 6,000 Americans die in home falls every year, according the Home Safety Council. That's an injury-to-death ratio of 333 to 1.)

Two issues that generalize to the world of work are raised by these figures. The first is that people tend to behave more safely when a task is dangerous. They are alert, switched on, situationally aware, and may even stop the task with a time out for safety (TOFS) dynamic risk assessment. In so many organizations, however, it's the simple everyday things that fill the accident books.

Second, the simple everyday things that cause the most problems have to do with one simple risk factor that we cannot design out, no matter how sophisticated our organization or society becomes. The risk factor that we simply cannot design out is *gravity*, and this raises its head in a variety of situations.

For example, a huge number of the 'clothing' accidents mentioned above relate to women *falling* off high heels. One case study from an oil company in the North Sea I worked with in the late 1990s is that they had 5 LTIs that year. Two were on the three rigs they operated in the North Sea, but three happened at head office, and all three were women employees in heels falling on stairs.

Because they are collated from different clinics and hospitals, it's impossible to be exact about figures and categorizations. It's easy to imagine clothing accidents covering dislocated shoulders, as well as the one horrible zip injury most men suffer – but typically just the once! Half-on trousers, like inappropriate or hazardous footwear, must overlap with trips I'd imagine. (I'll skip over jokes about half-on trousers and irate husbands and later explanations for facial injuries that start with 'I had a fall darling . . . '.) A practical example with a large commercial overlap would be the fact that motorbikes are so much more dangerous than cars simply because you can't fall off or be knocked off a car. (Here's a quick exercise: think of as many famous people as possible who had an accident that made the news. What percentage involved gravity?)

Regardless of categorizations, it's clear that gravity is implicated one way or another in the vast majority of personal incidents. Stairs are dangerous. Appropriate footwear is as advisable in an office and in an icy car park as it is on an oil rig. In short, no organization can possibly hope to achieve or strive meaningfully towards zero harm without a systematic and practical approach towards gravity-related issues. Regardless of whatever dismissive process safety engineers might say, we have to have organizations where people:

- step up and down squarely;
- walk mindfully, alert to trip hazards;
- hold handrails on stairs;
- maintain three points of contact on ladders;
- lift kinetically, using only big muscle groups squarely applied (no stretching or twisting);
- don't stand under things that might fall on them, unless it's unavoidable; and
- wear hard hats where appropriate.

This is not an exhaustive list, of course, but here's a simple example based on real data. In the offshore oil industry, the likelihood of falling down the stairs is only about 1 in 100,000, despite the stairs being steep, metal and often wet. Consequently, with luck and a following wind, workers may enjoy an entire career offshore never holding that handrail and never falling. More than that, the unlikelihood of a single act leading to an accident also gives managers an excuse for a dose of 'blind eye' syndrome, so as to avoid potential scorn and backchat. However, over the years, as many workers have been killed in falls offshore as were killed in the Piper Alpha disaster, and account for a huge percentage of LTIs every year.

It works like this. Stairs will be used about a million times a year on a typical platform, so if *nobody* holds the handrail we'll suffer 10 falls a year on average. If 90% hold the handrail, we'll suffer one a year on average.

However, if 99% hold the handrail, we'll see one every 10 years. And 'zero harm' (in terms of accidents at least) in a given year becomes viable.

Gravity, simple accidents, blame and inappropriate responses

Because all slips and falls seem avoidable, this is an area where blame easily attaches and best practice is easily ignored. One example is failing to apply the simple safety hierarchy of designing out the risk. The UK Health and Safety Laboratory gives an excellent example of a fatality at a nightclub that was investigated in depth only because there was suspicion that the man who died had been pushed down the steps by bouncers (doormen), rather than suffering a drunken fall.

From the off, it was apparent that these steep steps were a deathtrap. They were badly lit, with 'handrails' flush to the wall that were essentially decorative only, and with occasional steps of different heights promoting 'cat paw, air steps'. The accident book showed that falls and injuries were frequent and that this wasn't even the first fatality.

It's true that most users of these stairs were drunk at the time of their accidents, but instead of a fatalistic '*stuff happens*' approach, it's vital that we deal with this clear combination of risks proactively and, at the very least, get the basics right.

Another example: Metal escalators have a slat design that mirrors the original wooden materials but reduces the amount of available contact points and is visually confusing when stepping off. You'll note that stepping off such escalators is harder than stepping on. What people expect needs to take second place to the safest design.

Given the data suggesting that slips, trips and falls are public enemy number one, we should crowd the halls when an expert stands up to talk about the topic, but instead we snigger. Attacking Heinrich (or Bird) wholesale because of the predictive validity of the data collected is throwing a very important baby out with the bathwater. The principle holds in all aspects of life: music, chess, golf, mindfulness, safety, health and driving included.

Health & Safety Statistics 2008			
	Highways	Rail	Cost
Fatal	0	0	
Major	3	0	136500
3 Day	11	0	60291
Minor	99	0	207603
Hazards & Near Misses	21	683	
AFR (5.45)	3.2	0	
Days Lost	104	0	21736
No. of Employees	1558	202	
Hours Worked	2828907	525134	£426130

Figure 3.2 Client data showing the power of near miss reporting

Here's an example where the predictive validity of the data is hopeless. In one column, lots of data but no accidents, and in another lots of accidents but little predictive data – indeed, more a diamond than a triangle. It very clearly shows, however, that working systemically as far down the triangle as possible, what we can call the 'Heinrich principle' is effective.

Driving safety and new technology

Young drivers sit in the middle of a perfect storm of risk. They have brains that don't fully mature until they are in their early twenties, so they feel immortal. That may be useful for raising an infantry, but it is less than ideal when in charge of a ton of fast-moving metal. They are often socializing in what is a mobile youth club much of the time, and are frequently listening to loud music, which robs them of important road noise feedback. Worse, they are obsessed with what peers think of them.

It's a nightmare for any parent or fellow road user.

Therefore, the use of tachometers to measure sharp braking and allowing insurance companies to give direct and instant feedback to young drivers by upping or even cancelling insurance premiums is excellent behavioural safety practice. Sharp braking correlates better with accidents than speed because it also covers attention to the road and distance from others, which may reflect underlying issues such as fatigue. So we have a strong algorithm, feedback based on accurate measurement and consequences both positive (access to independent travel, cheaper costs) and negative (cost, loss of vehicle). Added to this, in most countries, we are 10 times more likely to lose a worker through an accident on the roads than in work. So this isn't just excellent 'behavioural safety'; it's also extremely cost-effective.

This is an excellent example of how new technology, cleverly applied, can enhance a BBS process. Palmtop technology allows for information dissemination, collation and illustration way beyond anything possible when I first put together a training course or a check-sheet. As we invent and perfect contact lenses that can monitor physiology and send warning messages to our computers, or even order a prescription to be waiting for us when we get home, the possibilities are mind-boggling.

Recently, as well as for coming up with innovations themselves, some companies have begun to give similar rewards to people who adopt the innovations of others. How extremely sensible! This is a best practice we recommend to all clients. Similarly, a good BBS process will always look to innovate and 'steal' with speed and pride.

I attend a lot of events as a speaker, and even as a panelist in a *Dragons' Den* style competition where suppliers compete to win 'best new innovation' awards. It's not a job I like, as I want everyone to win, and most seem deserving. I recently saw a new air filter that lets you know when it needs changing, some excellent easily portable lattice flooring for fragile roofs, hugely impressive-looking plastic adjustable and self-fixing barriers, tailored insoles made of a new shock-absorbent material to help with lower back pain, and lightweight wrap-around safety specs resistant to every sort of scratch, glare or temperature issue.

There are many practical answers to the question 'Why isn't everyone buying just about everything?' but it doesn't stop you asking it! There really are 'solutions' everywhere, often to problems I might not even know I had. Naturally, most come at a premium price, but none at a price that would put many off.

Well-being

In the UK, around five workers will kill themselves for every one we lose using the roads for work (so about 37 times the likelihood of them dying in an accident at work). The exact figures vary, but adjusting the stated ratio for talks in countries such as Ireland, the US and New Zealand recently was required not because suicide rates are dissimilar in these countries, but because UK workplace fatalities are relatively low. (134 UK fatalities at work last year compared to circa 5,000 suicides of working-age people.)

Therefore, the number of times a supervisor notices that a worker is unusually quiet or hyperactive and asks if they are OK, the better. The first thing you'll be taught on a mental health awareness course is to look for changes in behaviour. If we take a holistic view of harm and work from a data-driven perspective, then instigating such conversations is without any doubt the most important BBS behaviour any supervisor can possibly undertake. And it certainly helps build trust and enhance communication, both of which are central to a strong culture, as we know.

Indeed, incorporating resilience training, soft skills for supervisors and well-being creation programmes is essential to a holistic BBS approach for day-to-day safety reasons too. This is because stressed individuals are initially flooded with adrenaline as the 'fight or flight' response kicks in. In the short-term, adrenaline can be a good thing, sharpening reflexes and delivering energy. Over time, however, that adrenaline is replaced by a build-up of cortisol. This isn't good. High levels of cortisol typically makes people risk-averse and cautious, which is not entirely a bad thing from a safety perspective, but may not result in the most dynamic behaviour that companies want for growth.

Of more direct relevance is that people who are full of cortisol also often prove inattentive, panicky and impetuous:exactly what awareness-raising sessions exhort us not to be, and certainly not what we want of the pilot flying our plane or the driver of our bus.

Many well-being gurus stress that resilience is not about the person, but about the environment in which they find themselves, and doing something about it, if it involves task demands that are stressful. This might be the case because onerous task demands are stressing everyone. Alternatively, it could be because an individual has been given more autonomy than they are comfortable with. We build a strong supportive culture interaction by the interaction and objective analysis of such task demands.

These views are supportive of the central thrust of this book. Excellence is just excellence and overlaps. Much of the training and culture development I've suggested as key to a holistic BBS approach will, utterly inevitably, impact positively on well-being as well.

Summary

The Heinrich principle is universal and eternal. It applies to basic risk factors, such as the behaviours relating to gravity that account for the majority of accidents, but also to cultural factors that are more holistic, and which impact on well-being too.

Nearly every BBS approach comes with the boast, 'We say here it's OK to challenge and it's OK to be challenged'. This can't be bought off a shelf or even willed into truth. It has to be built, interaction-by-interaction.

Similarly, risk is reduced behaviour-by-behaviour, innovation-by-innovation. In the end, we get the rate of harm we *deserve* – everything else is names, details and case studies.

4   A lack of safety leadership

An acceptance of what constitutes the root cause of so many unsafe and risky behaviours and a commitment to objectively understanding what's going wrong (or a 'mindful' safety culture, as described by Andrew Hopkins) underpins everything that's good about behavioural safety.

Heinrich's infamous triangle fills up most readily not because of bad worker attitudes, but with the consequences of suboptimal leadership behaviours and thoughts. This is because a trip hazard is a trip hazard and a shortcut a shortcut, but a culture that tolerates trip hazards and shortcuts will typically also tolerate a lack of PPE, systems being negated, blind eye syndrome, and so on. The number one direct cause of unsafe behaviour is poor supervision.

It's a mindset issue. Do the organization's leaders see unplanned and unwelcome events as irritations or as learning opportunities? People who whine are telling you they are unhappy, and this is worth investigating. Sometimes you'll find they are just always unhappy, of course, but often they'll have a genuine grievance. (And even if it *is* them, we can instigate a review of the efficacy of our selection efforts!)

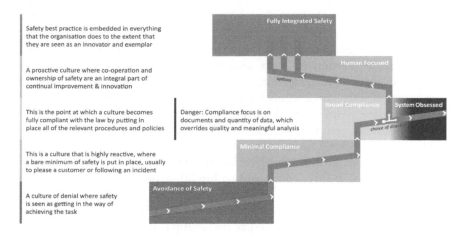

Figure 4.1 The Bizzell/Roscoe 'Fork in the Road' Culture Model

Senior leadership commitment

Most people agree that senior management commitment is as close to *everything* as makes little difference. I have seen BBS approaches flourish without it in the short- or even medium-term, but it's like batting on a poor wicket. No matter how well you are performing, it can all fall apart in an instant, as the foundations are not solid.

There isn't an experienced BBS consultant without stories of CEOs woodenly reading out a talk written for them by the head of HSE. A former colleague tells of a CEO popping his head around the door and asking him to prepare a talk that he could present the following week to demonstrate his commitment to HSE. Chief executives who can emote like Bill Clinton or Tony Blair may get away with it *on the day*, but not necessarily later.

Case studies

My worst experience is sharing a stage with the wonderful Jason Anker. Jason's testimony about paralysing himself in a simple and easily avoidable fall in 1993 is heartfelt, moving and brutally honest. (Jason's story is easily accessed on the Internet, or see Proud2bSafe at p2bs.org). Like the presentations of the US's Charlie Morecraft, who was badly burned in an accident in 1990 working for Exxon, it is 'once heard, never forgotten' and very humbling. He doesn't have to give anywhere near that much of himself to justify the fee.

A chief executive who had said all the right things in a wooden, slightly pompous, obviously *written-for-him* speech walked to a waiting car straight past Jason soon afterwards without a word of thanks. I won't tell you what I thought, but I will tell you it's not easy turning work down when you have wages to pay. We did in this case, and the SHE team who'd set the day up, and admitted privately to ongoing despair at this man's attitude, fully understood.

On another occasion, I worked with the board of a midsized food company whose charismatic CEO clearly had the rest of the board pretending to agree with his every word and not articulating the fact that they had reservations. We ran a session and made a plan. Although the CEO *did not* finish with the infamous rhetorical question 'So we're all agreed?' and then, after issuing a steady stare, asking for anyone disagreeing with him to show themselves, a sense of unease was palpable, and it was obvious that the rest of the senior team wanted something more simple or to delay any BBS approach for a while. It was, of course, an issue of competing demands and resources.

Three months later, I returned for a follow-up and found that the CEO had recently announced he was moving on and wouldn't be joining us. The session was instead hosted by his deputy, and within 30 seconds it was apparent that the project was effectively stone dead.

Early in my career, I spoke at a conference on 'Readiness for BBS' and took two clients with me as case studies. The first group from an oil company spoke about how the roll-out of an empowerment programme had primed them perfectly for the sophisticated and very successful process we implemented. While the first client was speaking, the second set of clients, from a pallet repair outfit, were smiling and laughing.

The first question when they took their turn was to ask what was so amusing about the oil company group. They explained that they were looking at the readiness slide the oil company referred to and felt that they didn't even qualify for rung one, let alone the penultimate one that the previous speakers felt they'd achieved.

Their story was a simple one. Their CEO and managing director had been to a funeral in the west of England to bury an employee who had been killed at work. Understandably devastated, they had stopped at a service station on their way back north and made a plan. It included deciding to never promote anyone who didn't hold a basic UK-based safety qualification and also to hire me, who they had come across at a London conference. I naïvely proposed a comprehensive BBS approach with safety committees writing their own items, time-intensive measurement schedules providing data to be used at workforce-run goal-setting sessions, and charts updated weekly. They went for five categories, each containing six items, a real logistical stretch for a company with some really aggressive production targets.

There was kickback from management at some sites, questioning whether the leadership really wanted this approach, but that didn't last beyond discovering they really *did*. Management, led by Neil S and Vince M, ably supported by Dave F and Wayne B, among others, drove it through. Forgive me the name check – I'll be grateful to these guys forever – they helped launch my career. Without their commitment, my inexperience would have led to the bullish methodologies I'd proposed falling flat on their face! As it was, a couple of years after the pilot site launched, they were able to show a reduction in accidents to one-tenth of the original levels. It made a stunning case study included in several Institute of Occupational Safety and Health (IOSH) publications.

In this case, developing ownership was an explicit aim of the methodology, and 20 years later they are still running a successful BBS programme, despite all the main players moving on, or in one case passing away. The oil company was indeed primed for great success, and the division we were working with won all sorts of awards – until its central office imposed a company-wide scheme based on a 'Type 3' methodology.

While this method stems from the principle that good safety is driven by line management on a day-to-day basis, it seldom empowers, and sometimes even alienates, workforces. In this case, it led to a severely demotivated workforce and the end of the scheme we'd set up.

Reason concludes *The Human Contribution* with the observation that 'safety is a guerrilla war, one that you will probably lose' eventually. We must fight a clever rearguard action as best we can for as long as we can. This is the essence of the reality of BBS and safety management, especially when we take a more in-depth and holistic look at the notion of 'zero harm'.

It's almost impossible to drive through medium- to long-term improvement without senior management commitment, but we need to help them by tailoring a methodology that maximizes workforce empowerment. Like a good guerilla army, we need to be astute, focused and flexible. We need to know what we're trying to achieve, why we're trying to achieve it, and what the strengths and weaknesses of our options are. We need robust but flexible plans with options and leeway built in.

Leaders, like everyone else in organizations, are hard-wired to do what they think will be best received. They are stuck in the middle, passing on problems that have been passed down to them. The term 'supervisor squeeze' covers it well. Everyone is looking up and looking for clues. The Just Culture perspective is merely a reflection of C-suite motivation.

This tends to reflect the personality of the key people and the CEO in particular. In my experience, many of the organizations with the strongest leadership are shaped in this way because of the personal experience of the CEO at a funeral. A mining company we worked for was transformed almost overnight when the CEO was approached by the widow of the worker whose funeral it was. He assumed he was going to get a mouthful of abuse or even a slap, but was moved when she thanked him for showing her husband the respect of attending, which he found very humbling. It utterly changed his mindset, and thereafter the approach of the whole company.

I've attended hundreds of annual safety days, and I'd say that the following four talks cover 99% of all those I've heard. They're important because of their correlation with the behaviour of front-line management:

1   A speech by a CEO clearly written for them by the SHE director and not at all convincing. Such speeches in my experience are nearly always followed by the CEO departing via a side door soon after the talk's delivery.
2   A talk by an articulate and intelligent CEO, written for them by the SHE director, saying all the right words and looking reasonably convincing.
3   A talk by a CEO based on a genuine appreciation that an investment in safety is an investment in general excellence and a 'win-win' for all concerned.
4   A talk by a CEO that stunned the room and was utterly convincing. As well as an appreciation of 'win-win', such speeches nearly always contain a powerful personal testimony about the funeral or death of a colleague.

I sometimes feel that the essence of what we do as safety consultants is simply to boost the number of 'type three and four' talks, so that real excellence is sought proactively, not reactively.

Leadership and learning

The best HSE writers stress that proactive thinking is key, and there are many who consider a learning focus to be central to the progress and development of mankind as a *species*. Books such as *Black Box Thinking* by Matthew Syed argue that times when defensive rationalizations are minimized correlate well with events such as the Reformation and the Enlightenment. A learning focus is not just good for organizations; it's good for us as a *species*.

When Galileo first suggested that the earth rotated around the sun, and not the other way around, it went down badly with the powers that be. He pointed out that, if the authorities cared to join him in his observatory, he had a powerful new telescope. If they looked through it, he could show them proof that his theories were right.

They declined and put him under house arrest for the rest of his life.

Andrew Hopkins, in *Failure to Learn*, stresses that the key element of a strong safety culture is that it be 'mindful'. What he means is that all organizations are full of problems and issues, but the best ones, mindful that this is true, proactively go out and find these problems. Weaker organizations, by contrast, wait passively for problems to find them. Applying Reason's analogy, there are lots of holes in the Swiss cheese, and identifying where and when these holes appear is key.

Under Just Culture, we discussed a number of issues that directly drive unsafe behaviour. Here, I'd like to cover a few fundamental reasons why a supervisor or manager might analyse a situation and come to an inaccurate conclusion as to what caused it.

My dear old Uncle John was a lovely man, but he did have the habit of pondering a situation, then announcing confidently, 'I think you'll find . . .'. Very often, he was utterly wrong, most infamously within our family when announcing with total certainty, 'I think you'll find this crisis will bring those two much closer together'. The duo in question, of course, never spoke to each other again.

The world is infinitely complex and becoming evermore so. To deal with this complexity, people use a variety of mental shortcuts, or 'heuristics', to help

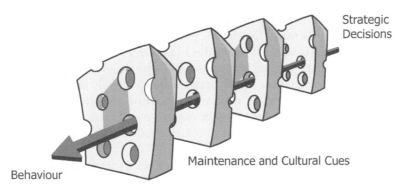

Strategic Decisions

Maintenance and Cultural Cues

Behaviour

Successive layers of defences, barriers, and safeguards

Figure 4.2 Reason's Swiss Cheese Model (Source: adapted from Reason 2008)

make sense of the world. Often, this is helpful. Indeed, it would be difficult to get to the end of a given day if we analysed everything completely from scratch. Sherlock Holmes, remember, didn't actually need to work for a living! Often, however, when we apply one of these heuristics we'll be wrong.

Some examples:

Planes are interesting toys, but of no military value.
                     (Marshal Foch, 1911, describing the French Air Force.
                                The Red Baron and others demurred.)

Who the hell wants to hear actors talk?
                                                (H.M. Warner, 1927)

There is a world market for maybe five computers.
                               (Thomas Watson, chairman of IBM, 1943)

You never win anything with kids.
                     (British soccer expert Alan Hansen at the start of
                        the 1995/96 Premier League season that ended
                            up being dominated by Sir Alex Ferguson's
                                       youthful Manchester United side)

Dire . . . clichéd . . . a disaster.
                     (Ian Main, light entertainment commissioner at the BBC,
                        1970s, when deliberating whether to commission the
                        first series of the iconic TV comedy series *Fawlty Towers*.
                           Indeed, he only did so because John Cleese, the
                                 lead writer, was already an established star.
                                     The programme continues to be voted the
                                          funniest situation comedy of all time.)

There are thousands of examples of people who are supposed to be experts in their field who just *got it wrong*. I haven't even mentioned the dozens of people who turned down J.K. Rowling, The Beatles and Harper Lee, because it's easy to do that in fields where 'no, no, and again no' is the *default* setting. Indeed, being *primed* to make a mistake is an important issue to actively watch out for.

We're diverting to this area of psychology because the most important building block of a strong BBS process is an objective understanding of what's happening and why. Get this wrong and all else that follows is likely to be a less than efficient use of resources.

So why do we convince ourselves that it's Sherlock Holmes looking back at us from the mirror when it's actually Homer Simpson? Some important issues have a direct impact on behavioural safety, either because they affect individual risk-taking or because of the way they are interpreted by colleagues. Incidentally, Arthur Conan Doyle, the author of Sherlock Holmes, might be considered the very definition of logical, and certainly articulates deductive reasoning extremely well in his books. In real life, he believed in fairies.

Let's start with a truth that undermines just about everything.

Your memory is largely fiction

Your memory is like a film archive comprised of things you saw, things you thought you saw, and even things you only imagined. Unfortunately, once these memories are in the archive, the labelling is so terrible that's it is very difficult or impossible to tell one from the other.

Here's a famous example. Please read and memorize the following list of words:

> door, glass, pane, shade, ledge, still, house, open, curtain, frame, view, breeze, sash, screen, shutter

At conferences, I ask members of the audience to stand up if they genuinely recall the word 'door'. This is the primacy effect as it's the first word on the list. I then ask if they recall the word 'shutter'. That's the recency effect as it's the last word. Then finally, they stay standing and win a book if they recall the word 'window'.

Of course, 'window' isn't in that list at all, it's just implied, but there are always several people claiming they have heard it.

In another well-replicated study, it was shown that you could vary the reported closing speed of a traffic accident depending on the words used to describe it, starting with 'when the two vehicles *touched*', then changing that to '*collided*' and ending with '*smashed into each other*'. The latter wording elicited a remembered speed that was 50% greater than the first.

So sometimes, even if you see an event with your own eyes and remember it clearly, you'll be less accurate in your interpretation than an eyewitness who saw it too, is able to channel Just Culture classifications like a sixth sense, and feels they understand the individual's motives behind it.

Some other causes of subjectivity and error:

Overconfidence

The only people with an accurate view of themselves are the clinically depressed. This bias is really helpful as we seek the confidence and optimism to take on an uncertain and often hostile world, but it doesn't do us many favours when we need to question whether our instinctive judgements are sound.

I have a decade-old slide based on notes taken from a talk at a Scottish road safety event by a policeman who quoted a study that found 48% of Scottish drivers thought they were average in ability and another 48% above average. More in-depth analysis of the remaining 4%, who at first glance had modestly labelled themselves as below average, found most confessing how their superb eye–hand coordination, lightning–sharp reflexes and extensive experience left them overconfident. Without a full reference, the quality of the study can't be verified, but we recognize the emotion I'm sure. Especially when an issue of self–esteem is on the line, the worst we'll rate ourselves is average. (Quick test: how good a *lover* are you?!) This esteem–protecting mindset is important, as when we make the point that 'some people really need to improve, and you know who you are', almost everyone is pointing at the person sitting next to them.

A personal example of overconfidence concerns the leader of a steelworks for whom we conducted a culture survey. Once the report was written, I gave feedback personally, and it wasn't good reading. On arrival, the CEO announced, 'I've decided we don't need the full report or the briefing, just the headlines. Just tell me who we need to shoot first'. He then detailed his exasperation with the feckless workers, who he was sure were half the time injuring themselves just so that they could claim compensation.

I explained that the first hour was an explanation as to why shooting any-one at all nearly always proves counterproductive, and how, when you point a finger at someone, three of your digits are pointing back at yourself. However, he insisted, 'I know about culture. Trust me'. It was good–natured banter, so I asked him to outline the principles underpinning ABC analysis, Just Culture or Reason's Swiss cheese model, all of which he'd find hugely useful as his company developed plans to drive forwards its safety culture.

Challenged like this, he snarled, 'Listen. I know all about what a strong safety culture looks like, believe me'. Before I could stop myself, I replied, 'Then you do the presentation and start with why you have such a crap one'.

This didn't cost us a long–term client, since one year after this exchange the parent company gave up entirely and closed the place. I imagine that the former CEO is still moaning that he had no chance of success, given the work-force he inherited. At least his laid–off steel workers had the benefit of no longer having to work in his miserable, badly led, blame–riddled factory.

Another story with no positive side benefit regales an argument I saw at a conference in Malaysia, where an 'I've seen it all' type was, fuelled with drink, ripping into his global SHE director about the 'elf and safety B*&^%s' he had been 'forced to travel halfway around the world to endure'.

The SHE director continued to calmly make the moral case for improve-ment, pointing out the unimpressive global accident and fatality rates. The executive responded that he wouldn't listen to such 'emotive crap'. He knew it all, having been emotionally affected by the funerals of three of his employees. He said this without irony, despite having been the site manager on each occasion.

The response he got was effectively, 'What a shame it is for your staff and their families that you even needed to go to one – let alone two more'.

We are all overconfident. It helps us get out of the front door with our heads up, but is unhelpful at nearly all other times. A simple data-driven exam-ple from the bestselling myth-busting book *Freakonomics* by Steven Levitt and

Stephen Dubner is that alcohol makes us overconfident, as well as impairing our senses, which doesn't help when people walk home drunk. This is statistically eight times more likely to lead to death than driving home drunk, yet few people who are killed are worried about their personal safety at the time.

Expectation and confirmation bias

We often see what we expect to see, and this doesn't help the innocent new recruit of a contractor with a bad reputation. They're motivated and conscientious, but committing unintentional errors, maybe because of a lack of training or because the company the contractor is carrying out work for gave a poor induction. However, management simply sees yet another example of a contractor's sloppy attitude to safety and simply fires off a blame-filled email.

Again, we need to put ourselves in their shoes, or, in Dekker's terminology, realize that both zigging *and* zagging would have looked perfectly acceptable. It is only experience that shows us zagging was the wrong choice.

You're probably guilty of this too. A simple example: Do you feel that everyone driving slower than you on the motorway is a 'wuss' while everyone driving faster is a maniac?

Another simple example that illustrates how we are hard-wired to see what we expect to see, and then seek proof to confirm it, is a card trick described by UK 'mentalist' Derren Brown to set people up to learn from a simple failure. To do this, he lays out four cards on a table and explains that each card has either the letter A or the letter D on one side and either the numbers 3 or 7 on the other:

A   D   3   7

He explains that if there is an A on one side, then there will be a 3 on the other, and the challenge is which cards need to be turned over to see if

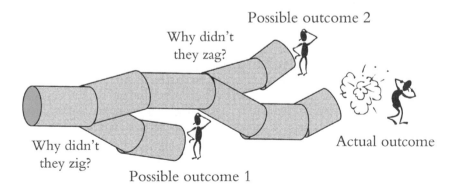

Figure 4.3 Hindsight Model (Source: adapted from Dekker 2006)

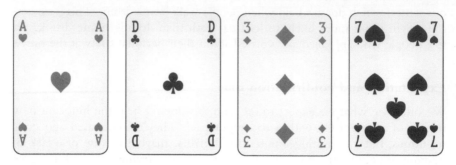

Figure 4.4 Seeking confirmation of established belief, card example

that's true. Under time pressure, most people will go for turning over one A and one 3 card.

The actual answer is A and 7. You do need to turn over A, as, if there isn't a 3 on the back, the rule is disproved. However, whether there is an A or a D on the back of the 3 doesn't double-check whether there are also rules that say that the D must have a 3, 7 or nothing at all. However, if we turn over the 7 and find an A on the other side, *it disproves the rule.*

To paraphrase Nassim Nicholas Taleb's book *The Black Swan*, about unlikely but devastating incidents, if I see a million white swans it does not prove that all swans are white. But if I see just one black swan, it's proof positive that not all swans are white.

Using this principle means that we must fight away confirmation bias by always critically challenging assumptions, especially our own. Similarly, when going into a debate or negotiation, it's a good idea to not just think of my strengths and your weaknesses, but to force yourself to think also of my weaknesses and your strengths.

Studies show that expectation bias can be really powerful so that we actually experience what we expect to. Told that one wine is classy and expensive and that a second is cheap plonk, though both are exactly the same, the pleasure centre of the brain lights up more for the 'expensive' wine. This isn't lying to look sophisticated. It actually does taste nicer merely because you expected it to. A second example is the balsamic vinegar in beer test. It enhances the flavour but isn't always added as it's far more expensive than beer. Told that a beer has had an expensive flavour added, most people will agree that this has been beneficial. In contrast, if they are informed that, unfortunately, while they were away some vinegar was been spilled into their beer but that it will actually taste nicer as a result, most will disagree violently.

This combines with overconfidence so that, for example, a time-poor manager who reviews an incident badly and ticks the 'individual violation' box when they shouldn't do so doesn't just think he is right. He *knows* he is right.

Primal fears

Almost entirely subconscious motives also cause unsafe behaviour. The primal fear of letting down our tribe, becoming obsolete and being pushed outside of the cave into the snow underpins much of what's best about human behaviour – notions such as fairness, cooperation and trust.

Stress will often be triggered when we know job cuts are likely or where we are doing a job for which we haven't been properly trained. When we are anxious over long periods, we're not aware that we're full of cortisol or of the impact it's having on our day-to-day behaviour and health.

However, subconscious primal fears can influence our behaviour in other ways. For example, after the 9/11 terrorist attacks, so many people switched from planes to cars in the US that an *extra* 3,000 people died on America's roads the following year. The motivating fear of being wiped out by a rival 'tribe' actually hastened a different tragic consequence.

Similarly, if we stand on a beach underneath a coconut tree and see a shark fin in the water, perhaps the greatest primal fear of all – being eaten alive by a predator – will send a shiver down most spines. Yet, every year, more than 10 times as many people are killed by falling coconuts as by sharks.

We also appear to massively overreact to virus scares such as SARS or bird flu, but that's hard-wired too, and with good reason. Consider the impact of early European explorers on the Americas with the germs they brought with them. In the last century alone, more people were killed by the Spanish flu that swept the world just after World War I than in the war itself.

This isn't a reminder about the perils of overusing antibiotics, though that really *should* worry us as a species, but a lead-up to saying that we always need to strive for a mindful analysis of what we're doing and why we're doing it. We need objective analysis and data if our reasoning and actions are to be logical and proportional. We also need objective data to confirm we were correct. (analyse, measure, check). The mindset trap we must avoid is that our behavioural data isn't a confirmation that the workers are being less foolish and risky; it's confirmation that management know what they're doing.

Sunk costs

A man sits in a corner clicking his fingers every 10 seconds. Asked why he's doing it, he says that it keeps the killer elephants away. Told there are no killer elephants in the area, he replies that it is working – and carries on.

One of the biggest mistakes we make is to be led by sunk costs. Finding it difficult to admit you've made a mistake can lead to all sorts of bad habits, risky behaviour and unhelpful mindsets. It basically means being unable to deal with the fact that doing X now means admitting that the time you spent doing Y was wasted.

Cult organizations use this all the time with techniques such as 'flirty fishing'. This is where an attractive person will be sent out to approach someone of the opposite gender looking less than happy and offer them friendship along with a coffee and biscuit with 'no obligation'. Then a suggestion to drop in tomorrow, read a pamphlet, take a certain test or come on a wonderful retreat will follow. As the time, effort and opportunity cost of doing other things mounts up, people are drawn in. In time, they may end up quitting their jobs, giving cults all their money and denouncing their loving families.

No cult member was ever asked to do that first up!

On a more everyday level, the 'we've always done it this way' and 'not invented here' syndromes can block innovation and development. A skill all BBS consultants learn is that where an in-house team has cobbled something together that works 'okayish', you cannot dismiss it as 'okayish'. Without their time and effort, you'd have nothing to build on. If the team all quit, you'd be in real trouble, so any good consultant will work under the banner of 'evolution', even if it is actually more of a revolution.

Rewarding managers for implementing the good ideas of others, as well as for coming up with an innovation themselves, is excellent behavioural safety.

The fundamental attribution error (FAE)

Errors are all around us, and frequently in the thinking of those who analyse and judge the behaviour of employees and the causes of that behaviour. People aren't necessarily lying, being awkward or deceiving themselves. Regardless, it makes objectivity difficult.

Consider the following common error, which has a direct importance to the Just Culture principle and the methodologies that flow from it.

The FAE approach, as described by Lee Ross in 1977, says that we are hot-wired to judge an event overly critically to the person and underplay the role of the environment, unless the 'person' is us, in which case we overplay the environment and have all sorts of excuses for what we've done. Complicating matters further, the more serious the consequence of the behaviour, the more prone we are to make this error.

For example, you're driving along and suddenly in the mirror an irate driver is shaking their fist at you as you realize you've cut them up and come close to running them off the road. Most people will respond with the following rationales:

'Sorry, but you were in my blind spot/my partner borrowed the car and adjusted the mirrors and I forgot to move them back/if you knew how tired I was, what a rush I'm in or how upset and distracted I am, you'd understand/ there's no harm done so steady on . . . and there's certainly no need for *that*'.

Now consider a similar situation, only this time it's you that's nearly run off the road by someone driving a red sports car while speaking on a mobile phone. Five minutes later, you come around a corner to see them stood unharmed at the side of the car that they just wrapped around a lamppost and *still* on the phone. How many of us would laugh like a drain or even slow down and wind the window down to make a choice observation or two?

But how about this: you stop the car and wind the window down, but before you can make an observation you hear that the driver is a doctor rushing to an emergency and taking directions and giving emergency advice as they drove. They are now panicking, close to tears. Instead of issuing abuse, would you not switch to responding, 'Quick, get in. I'll drive you there'?

Consequences

Once things have gone badly wrong and there are consequences, it's difficult, if not impossible, to recover from this instinct to blame and punish.

For example, take the UK driver Gary Hart, who stayed up all night in Internet chat rooms, fell asleep at the wheel, and crashed off a road and down an embankment, finally coming to a halt on a train track at Selby, Yorkshire, in 2001. The next train along derailed and 10 people were killed. The driver was prosecuted and sentenced to five years in prison. The popular consensus was that he 'got off lightly', and there was a lot of criticism when he was released on probation after three years.

It didn't help that he refused to accept any blame for driving while so tired and ascribed the blame to 'fate'. But, even as we dismiss this bloke's self-justifying rationale and insulting nonsense, it's also worth asking ourselves how many of us have fallen asleep at the wheel. Thankfully, it's usually really briefly and consequence-free, but it's often because we stayed up late the night before, and not always working. Again, it's far more effective to deal with the risk by proactively analysing the extent and cause of drowsy driving, which we know to be extremely dangerous.

Case study: the Hillsborough disaster

If you ask what risk factors I might associate with a large sporting event, I would, as a layman, make a list including terrorist attacks, crush issues associated with a large number of people arriving late because of travel problems or direct from a last quick drink in the bar, and perhaps the need to segregate different fans in case of fighting. Looking at that list, you wouldn't think me particularly skilled or perceptive – they are all very obvious to anyone who's ever been to such an event.

However, after the Hillsborough tragedy in which 96 people were crushed to death, highly experienced police officers in charge of crowd safety denied any culpability, claiming, among other things, that it wasn't their fault as many supporters had turned up at the last minute, many of them drunk. Then, they orchestrated a cover-up along the lines of: 'They were just horrible working-class football fans on the beer but we're *police officers* – it stands to reason that the entire fault lies with them'.

Leadership, trust and discretionary effort: a summary

A simple learning point for behavioural safety practitioners is that the more proactive we can be in analysing why risky behaviours are occurring before anything serious happens, the better. Go further on down the line and it becomes a tennis match of blame, with lawyers, distortion, denial, projection, hindsight bias and good old-fashioned ass-covering.

A key component of the fabled 'interdependent' safety culture is 'brother's keeper' behaviours, also known as prosocial or 'citizenship' behaviours. I'd argue that all world-class safety cultures demonstrate an abundance of these, but you have to earn them the hard way.

Simon 'Leaders Eat Last' Sinek highlights the phrase 'I did it for them as I know they would have done it for me', and stresses that good leaders make a person feel safe because the relationship with them is underpinned by *trust* rather than fear, and the belief that when things go awry the reaction is to *help* and *coach* rather than to *blame*.

Deep in our psychology is that it is, always has been and always will be to an extent 'us against them'. Some 50,000 years ago, it was our tribe or hunting group against the world: nature, predators and hostile tribes. It's literally as basic and primeval as saying, 'I can't recover my strength by sleeping well if I can't trust you to take your turn on watch'. 'Us' in the modern world is the organization, the shift, the team or just the workmate who rides alongside you in the van or car.

I was once asked by a leading research house how they might deal with a problem a South American client had set them – getting workers to report other workers for breaches of rules that were not critical but were still relatively important. Was this something to do with South American culture? I replied that this was a generic issue and they were facing entirely the wrong direction. Such reporting of infractions that are only reasonably important simply never happens, except in highly fractious and politicized organizations with no cohesion at all that are frankly imploding. You don't ever turn on your teammate, if you can possibly avoid it.

I suggested a far better use of resources was to ask why breaches of rules occur, with no names, and no pack drill, just analysis-seeking solutions.

Being in charge is one thing, but being an effective leader is another. You'll have heard the saying that 'leaders have followers and good leaders have willing followers'. First, your team has to trust you to 'have their backs' if they are to be frank, open and give discretionary effort. They simply won't trust you if they don't think you're *just*. So, another reason why a well-designed and impartially administered Just Culture framework is so incredibly important is that it increases trust, transparency, consistency and fairness. This leads directly to objectivity of analysis and efficacy of response.

90% of the time when a worker dismisses their supervisor as a 'd*&^head', what they mean is that they perceive that the supervisor consistently fails to make an effort to empathize and support. Instead, the various faults from which we all suffer run unchecked and blame is abundant.

Section II

Behavioural safety solutions

Everything is interconnected

Everything contributes to safety culture, including the way individuals are selected, developed and retained. It starts in the pub when a newspaper advert is read or when a job opportunity is discussed. One of the most influential psychology papers of them all is Schneider's ASA theory, which says that certain people will be *attracted* to an organization, while others will be *selected*, and there will also be selective *attrition*.

Imagine a safety-oriented A* candidate in an interview with a company with a dubious safety and worker welfare reputation. If they are asked solely about productivity and profit by a panel, this will confirm the reputation, and they are likely to accept instead a similar financial offer from a more enlightened organization. If they do join and realize it is as bad as they feared or find they can't make the changes they hoped they could, they will be likely to move on far more quickly than we'd like.

In addition to basic reward and recognition issues, even the wording of a job specification contributes to the safety culture.

So when we run the most wonderful individual development and selection centres, we should make sure there are some safety and well being creation themes in those tabletop exercises. Constantly setting the right tone and throwing the right shadow is as important as challenging unsafe acts on a day-to-day basis, starting with the fact that there will be fewer unsafe acts to challenge.

Section II

Behavioural safety solutions

5   Planning for behavioural safety

What we need is to make a practical and viable plan, and ensure through monitoring that we see it through to fruition. This might be referred to as 'governorship', and there are 1,001 variations on this theme. Something systemic and holistic is required as a framework, and the one used by BST is included here.

Most BBS processes will include some version of a guiding committee, including safety or other shop-floor representatives, experts and line management. Often a dedicated project manager or 'champion' will be designated with, ideally, some combination of the two.

If the designated champion is someone about to leave or who has been transferred sideways several times to somewhere considered quiet and unimportant, we really need a committee.

What we are describing here is basic change management: plan, do, review and replan. It's no more complicated than turning a genuine desire for change into some sort of logical plan, then assessing systematically how well that plan is working out. 'Our aim is zero accidents as all accidents are preventable' is fine as a *principle*, but if that's all supervisors get told it's simply not going to happen. Likewise, a workforce left in tears by a moving personal testimony of somebody who has been injured at work is primed to do something 'better', but simply saying, 'Think on, take care and don't be like this man' is far too vague.

Lists should never be longer than five items, so, though using his terminology, Kotter's famous eight-stage change management model can be boiled down to:

- Establish that there is a need.
- Create a guiding coalition to develop and communicate a vision and strategy.
- Empower employees for broad-based action while generating short-term wins.
- Consolidate gains.
- Anchor new approaches in the culture.

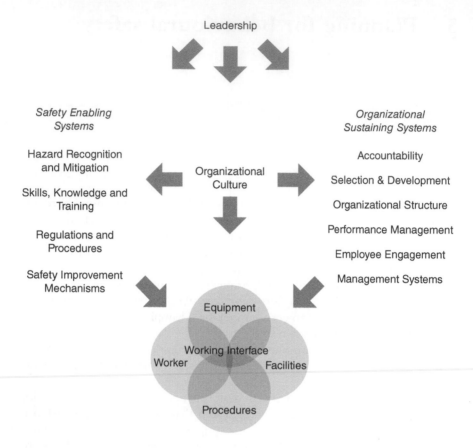

Figure 5.1 BST's holistic framework

We might cross-reference this approach with something as simple as a SMART goal to give us a robust plan. SMART has various versions, but mine is specific, measurable, agreed, realistic, reviewed and time-set.

First, what specifically are we aiming to achieve? Perhaps a reduction in accident rate from 2.0 to 1.0? This might be needed for morale reasons because someone has just got hurt and we must address a collective desire that something must be done to prevent that happening again. Or perhaps it's for business reasons as a major client is *demanding* that we describe a realistic plan for substantial improvement. Ideally, it'll be because the organization has chosen to proactively deliver a win-win, but that's the third most frequent reason on this short list, and even then it's usually on the back of the arrival of a new CEO.

Cynicism aside, whatever the motivation for halving numbers of incidents, it's great. In my experience, it's something that can realistically be achieved in one to two years, or sooner if conditions are favourable. Halve it again, then a *third* time over about five years, and you have a case study to grace any website or book. If that sounds simple, that's because it is, but countless organizations have achieved it and yours can too.

A practical plan will include a road map, developed ideally by a strategy team made up of operations, HR, HSE and union or shop-floor representation that comes up with something as simple as:

- Training all management and supervisors in 'risk literacy' and 'soft skills' over six months.
- Setting up a formal 'walk-and-talk' approach that allows these skills to be used on the H&S topic on a weekly basis.
- Embedding these new skills through an HR-run 360-degree follow-up formal appraisal, as well as informal day-to-day discussions and assessment using hand-held check-sheets.
- Including an element of coaching to support people as they try out their new skills.
- Training several BBS workforce teams tasked with analysing a handful of problematic behaviours of their choice and coming up with high-impact, low-cost solutions, as well as high-impact, high-cost solutions.
- Publicizing the changes that flow from these teams to maximize the opportunities for praise and to create a 'can-do' atmosphere (Kotter's short-term wins).
- Generating volunteers for a peer-to-peer 'walk-and-talk' approach, which may or may not involve measurement, as is appropriate.
- Inviting these volunteers to form a committee that will give itself a name (for ownership purposes) and control data monitoring and feedback processes.

This list is a solid top-down *and* bottom-up design that covers all Kotter's points. There are of course many variations on it. For a start, towards the end, it assumes a reasonably static and accessible workforce, such as you'd find in a factory. However, since your process is going to be based on *analysis* and *empowering leadership*, then something holistic and systemic will be entirely possible regardless of the challenges.

Ideally, we'll incorporate some metrics, starting with 'happy sheets' about the training courses, but it's really not rocket science. Work through these reasonably well and you'll have your step change in safety guaranteed.

A few strategic decisions are worth outlining here, since we're talking about overview strategy and it's difficult to distinguish between what's effective and what's symbolic as process and management commitment intertwine. For example, when volunteer teams come up with some 'high-impact, low-cost' ideas, put them into action. They will directly improve safety performance. However, maximizing the publicity associated with the changes helps create a feel-good factor that will increase the number of volunteers for anything else you're planning to do. It also motivates the original volunteers to go out and find *other* ideas. It's a virtuous circle of building trust and traction, driven by management commitment.

Essential and desirable elements when designing a safety framework (especially for an international roll-out)

If an organization has a very decentralized approach, then applying a highly centralized strategy will hit resistance, no matter what. However, while local ownership is always a good thing, there are a few key factors that must be the bedrock of any strategy, no matter how decentralized we'd like it to be. Specifically, here are three 'essentials' requiring a formal plan and associated rationale, regardless of where in the world you're working:

- *Learning*: How will the process maximize the objective understanding of why unwanted events are occurring? Answers will differ around the globe, but the more objective the understanding, the more likely that the chosen response will work.
- *Transformational leadership*: How will the local organization enhance and support the 'soft skills' such as coaching that maximize the number of 'willing followers' and the associated discretionary effort? Transactional leadership has an upper limit far below what we'll ideally be aiming for.
- *Empowerment and ownership*: Implemented well, the two issues above will automatically enhance this area. If we coach well and lead well, generally this will lead to workforce empowerment. However, we can also empower directly by delegating control of some aspects of the safety process; for example, setting up a committee with a budget that can be applied as it sees fit to any suggestion it generates, even an expensive one that's ratified by management as cost-effective.

Measurement

This is extremely useful for orientation and tracking, which enhances learning, and also for feedback using data and illustration as an element of coaching best practice. But it's on my desirable list, as doing it well is always difficult, and in some cases impossible, such as with peripatetic workers.

What we want is an informed and thoughtful decision as to what measurement will look like and how it will be used, if it is to be used at all.

What we don't want is a thoughtless acceptance or rejection of a methodology because everyone else is doing it, because it looks difficult or because head office bought a really expensive bit of software and everyone has to use it.

6   Identifying risks and pitfalls

Cultural measurement

Many organizations will measure their safety culture as an upstream cross-reference to the accident figures. We have one based on the Parker and Hudson (P&H) model with an essence of 'interdependence' added. BST use the Organizational Culture Diagnostic Instrument (OCDI). Both are based on sound research and have excellent predictive validity. There are many others on the market. My experience is that the vast majority of our clients are broadly *compliant* and wish to be broadly *proactive* as they strive towards a vision of world-class excellence (defined as 'generative' in the P&H model), so the core of this model really fits well as a reference point.

Whichever is chosen, an organization should remeasure a year or so later to check progress. These measures can be hugely useful, especially where there may be some resistance and defensiveness to overcome. Sometimes a CEO will be convinced that improvement is needed, and will commission a survey with which to hit his or her defensive management team over the head. A weaker position is where an HSE team will commission a survey to wave in the direction of the only half-convinced C-suite.

Sometimes an organization has a culture of measurement and will simply not take the subject area seriously if there are no measures in the system. To an extent, then, it's a *political* decision as much as a strategic decision as to whether cultural measures are used, but even a basic, hand-held, down-and-dirty measure is useful as a cross reference.

Accident figures can be understated and can even *increase* as the safety culture and its reporting improves, so it helps give a more accurate and rounded picture of what's really going on. It also helps with the 'measurable' and 'reviewed' element of any SMART approach.

I've had CEOs say, 'I don't need a survey. I know things need to improve significantly, so just make it so'. As management commitment to an ongoing process is *the* key, this isn't an insurmountable obstacle to success, and it's their money after all. Measurement, however, is a key element of nearly all good change management approaches (see Kotter, Six Sigma, *et al.*). Skipping it can prove a false economy.

Vision statement

A CEO might launch a branded safety process by standing up at an annual safety day and reading out a 'letter' written to him or her five years from now with the head of the safety representatives detailing the successful journey they've been on together and how proud they are to have halved accidents, then halved them again despite some initial scepticism.

Certainly, it's a bit corny, but if the commitment to achieving it is genuine, then it's worth it. It's only *not* worth it if the CEO is just mouthing words written for him or her by the director of HSE because everyone in the audience will know that's what they're doing and it'll be counterproductive.

It's the same with the 'storytelling, consultant-inspired' branding of a process. If, under that brand, a series of essential and desirable methodologies are selected, tailored and followed up systemically, then branding is a good idea. However, if it's just a hotchpotch of international randomness, then it's just likely to both bring the 'corporate meddlers' into disrepute and hinder local ownership.

Target Zero

Many organizations have adopted the Target Zero aim and logo as part of a BBS approach, and often this proves controversial. This doesn't need to be so if we see it not as an absolute target, but as an inviolate principle, namely that all accidents are preventable and none inevitable. Certainly, if we consider an organization of 20,000 or more people worldwide, someone, somewhere slipping over at the very least does seem close to inevitable, especially if the company had 145 LTIs the previous year. If there's a Target Zero for a year and it is missed in January, for example, workers may respond by thinking that they might as well all give up.

What the principle of Target Zero uses is the process of anchoring, as described by Kahneman and other writers on influencing skills. Here's how that works to paraphrase an example in *Thinking Fast and Slow*:

> Was Gandhi over or under 90 years old when he was killed?

> Was Gandhi older or younger than JFK when he was killed?

The first question anchors you to an older age than the second, as you start your deliberations and it significantly impacts on the figure you give for how old he was when he was killed. (He was 78 when he was shot.)

As the joke goes, 'For this year, we have a target of just one fatality and 25 LTIs. Who wants to volunteer?'

There's a wonderful scene in the 2001 Ken Loach film *The Navigators*, based on the UK rail industry. A 'going through the motions', ineffective junior manager is briefing his catcalling and jeering workforce about forthcoming changes. His talk includes the observation 'and safety has to improve too – we have a target of just two fatalities this year', in a tone that suggests that the third person who manages to get themselves killed will be in real trouble with senior management.

Target Zero is also especially controversial when applied to accidents of harm, partly due to the difficulty of definition. In the UK, for every employee killed at work, 18 will die on the roads in work-related travel. Worse than that, 45 people of working age will commit suicide. Suicide is usually a combination of issues: health, including mental health; family and friends; work and finances. If we only ascribe one-third of the causes to work, using Heinrich's principle, we can see that unsatisfactory work experiences contribute to the quiet desperation of millions on a daily basis. Then we need to get to the really awful data and consider the fact that around 100 people die of work-related illness due to exposure, for every one accident fatality. There may be a lag of decades or more, but can we really claim there's been 'zero harm' because we've had a year without an LTI?

This is a book arguing for a holistic and data-driven approach, so the mindset that no harm of any kind is inevitable is fine, indeed highly desirable. However, pushing it to anything more simply doesn't stand up to any sort of scrutiny. Setting an unrealistic target is a bad idea, but anchoring on excellence is a very good one.

Financial incentives

Incentives are very much a double-edged sword as they clearly demonstrate in a profound way that we all understand that safety is important to an organization. However, they can produce under-reporting in order to achieve targets and trigger bonuses. Some suggest that paying for safety like this sends an unhelpful message that safety isn't important for its own sake. On balance, I disagree, and feel that from this symbolic perspective, the benefit of symbolizing its importance with hard cash outweighs any such negative symbolism. It's not that safety isn't important for its own sake; it's just that having that in the heart of every one of our managers is, in 99% of organizations, an ideal we are currently *aiming* for. To paraphrase Bob Dylan 'Money doesn't talk, it swears' – but it swears *loudly*.

To be provocative, I wonder if half the organizations claiming that financial incentives for safety behaviour are 'unhelpful symbolically' are simply rationalizing a way of not having to swear loudly with hard cash and demonstrating that it's not something they consider important enough to 'pay' for.

Few have the same qualms when it comes to productivity.

What is utterly vital, however, is that for those of us who feel *learning* is the key to everything good, incentives do not compromise *reporting* in any way. This is achieved simply by three things:

- maximizing the amount of symbolic rewards reflecting genuine commitment to safety;
- cross-referencing any metrics with quality as well as quantity; and
- focusing as much as possible on process, rather than outcomes.

We need to directly reward behaviours associated with the quality of the learning, leadership and empowerment building blocks of a strong culture. For example, a safety element of a bonus might be triggered not by an absence of accidents or by an *apparent* absence, but by ensuring that supervisors undertake a suitable number of *good-quality* conversations about safety.

How many they can do can be fudged in the back of a van, but if we cross-reference that with some sort of 360-degree review of quality, you need a company-wide conspiracy. Let's stay sceptical and say that's still possible, but at this point it's just as easy to get on and just do it, so we're back in ABC theory territory.

Joined up

Good behavioural safety is holistic, so the first issue to address from a strategic point of view is how it dovetails with older approaches and more mainstream HR initiatives. Training in soft skills will incorporate all sorts of behaviours that directly or indirectly impact on all aspects of the organization. Even risk-literate thinking skills can, in nearly all cases, be readily applied to productivity. The Heinrich principle is not safety-specific, and even the Swiss cheese model, which describes multiple layers of protection from harm spliced with 'Five Whys' analysis, can be readily applied to everyday issues such as parenthood. Likewise, the 'soft' psychological benefits of a 'walk-and-talk' approach generalize. Safety may be the specific topic of conversation, but we cannot avoid building a culture where communication and empathy flourishes. You never hear an organization say, 'We've built a culture where it's OK to challenge and it's OK to be challenged, but only about safety'.

Therefore, the more a strategic plan acknowledges this 'interconnected and overlapping' truth and maximizes economies of scale, the better. HR and SHE squabbling over budgets, 'turf' and egos is not excellence.

Time spent ensuring that any new training course dovetails with and references previous courses and uses as much of its terminology as possible will not be wasted. It will also be appreciated by delegates.

In an ideal world, SHE and HR will work together and, in my experience, a follow-up meeting with the heads of both that goes well following a C-suite briefing nearly *always* correlates with a successful project. I once had a head of HR and training at a major company wait for us to be alone at a coffee machine and literally *hiss*, 'If you effing think you or your safety friends will ever do any training in this organization that's more than mere hazard-spotting, you're effing deluded'. She turned back to the room, smiling. You could base an entire module of a psychology degree on the debrief session of the subsequent pilot course that was hosted jointly by SHE and HR. Leading questions and subjectivity were the least of it. It was a cross between a game of tennis, a Freudian convention and the shoot-out at the O.K Corral.

If the HR and SHE is the *same person*, this either simplifies or complicates matters!

Discipline

Just because we are working from a Just Culture principle does not mean that discipline has no place in safety. Though a Just Culture analysis will *nearly always* show a factor more complex than wilful disregard for someone's own or a colleague's safety, there are times when it is appropriate.

An example might be a pilot with a drink problem who chooses to hide it rather than open up and take advantage of an in-house treatment scheme. We can empathize and understand that their brains might be scrambled by their addiction, *but* . . .

Or consider the worker who rushes to finish on time to get off and away to their second job. A key root cause might be an appallingly low hourly rate and children to feed, *but* . . .

In both cases, this has to stop.

In my experience, it's nearly always a grey area, even when discipline is clearly required. The trick is to use a systemic Just Culture decision tree model that maximizes objectivity and minimizes subjectivity. Dekker, in the book of the same name, among others, stresses that this matrix must be *written* and *administered* in conjunction with someone sympathetic to the worker (i.e. a union rep) to help prevent a drift to the status quo.

The key principle is to work as proactively as possible to ensure the need for the use of discipline is minimized. It's just hardly ever black and white when we're reacting, because once we're reacting, we're almost inevitably talking about blame, self-preservation, politics and making lawyers rich.

Unhelpful local culture and/or the socio-economic situation

A good cultural reference point would be films such as *Slumdog Millionaire* (2008), about underprivileged people in Mumbai, India, or *City of God*, a 2002 film about street gangs in the slums of Rio de Janeiro. A challenge often raised when designing a process is that, in some countries, the prevailing culture, or perhaps more specifically the background attitude towards individual risk, varies considerably.

That said, I do wonder if there is such a thing as a 'risk-*intolerant*' country. Risk tolerance is a universal trait that has helped us evolve from cave-living, and which every BBS programme ever implemented has had to address.

Happily, the reverse of the 'if the culture is wrong, then it doesn't matter about the system' problem applies. If the culture *within* the fence is right, then the mindset of an individual worker, regardless of where or how it is acquired, will have minimal impact, and we can have a strong and safe environment regardless.

Our BBS approach may need tailoring, but that's all. It always needs tailoring anyway. For example, there will be pockets of socio-economic micro-cultures in any country or organization, such as the bread-making factory in East

London controlled in part by management and in part by the 'uncle' who speaks little English and whose official job title is caretaker.

In short, it's your factory, and regardless of whether it's in India, Brazil or anywhere else, the culture on-site is largely yours to determine. Countless case studies from a whole range of consultancies and organizations have demonstrated the truth of this assertion. The catchment area from which you draw your workforce is simply no excuse.

One specific local problem can be cultural deference where a reluctance to say 'no' or to question a figure of authority can compromise the flow of information, analysis and communication. This was tackled directly by Korean Airlines when a co-pilot's last words just before his captain flew the plane into a mountain were, 'Er . . . excuse me captain sir . . . are you sure you're entirely happy about our altitude?' The last time he'd had the temerity to question the captain's authority, he'd been given a slap. The airline tackled this successfully with assertion training and having English as the cockpit language, to overcome the natural deference of the Korean language.

Such situations need systemic thought and methodologies to circumvent this cultural problem. Specifically, we need to use methodologies that focus on depersonalizing situations. So we should utilize assertion training indeed, as the airline did, but also proactively use depersonalized, entirely *analysis*-based questions such as 'What are people tempted to do?' Even in the most deferential 'what happens in Vegas stays in Vegas' situation, workers will talk about what *other* workers are *tempted* to do. Dropping people 'in it' rarely happens *anywhere*, but everyone likes an opportunity to contribute and show they understand something if there are no potential negative consequences.

The fact that many colleagues live in shacks with intermittent electricity and travel to work on some of the world's most dangerous roads is just a variation on a theme. You never hear an organization say, 'Well, a parts failure rate of 30% isn't too bad when you consider that's on a par with the electrical supply to the typical flat or house of most of our front-line workers'.

They shouldn't say it about safety either.

Home safety

Increasingly, organizations are taking the view that a colleague's safety outside the workplace should be of concern. Some are even actively censorious about this, so much so that some sort of official punishment would follow should you injure a toe trimming the grass in sandals or falling from a height because of inappropriate access.

An organization needs a very strong safety culture to get away with that, and in my view it requires a very strong and *overly paternalistic* culture that will almost certainly have unintended consequences in terms of generating limited amounts of discretionary effort. I just can't imagine an organization where punishing a worker for a home accident would fit with the most effective overall culture and holistic strategy. It would also suggest a certain overconfidence.

The use of positive techniques, especially around 'nudge' theory, are nearly always appropriate, however. A 'toolbox talk' on the vital importance of tyre wear and pressure using data and illustration, followed by the gift of a tyre pressure and tread depth checker, is clearly appropriate. Data- and illustration-based 'toolbox talks' followed by fire blankets for kitchens, carbon monoxide alarms and eye protection for gardeners who use power tools, given out 'with love and without prejudice', are also to be applauded. Then there are safety gates for new parents, because hardly any children put their fingers in sockets but lots fall down the stairs.

Some people may be cynical and sneering about such paternalism. This, I'd like to suggest, is one of those times when it's appropriate to think, "*Forget* you!"

Where it can be tricky is with issues such as 'grey fleets'. In some countries, an employer will be liable should something go wrong, and their efforts to ensure this doesn't happen are insufficient. We had a client where tyre pressure checkers were given out and a 'toolbox talk' was given, along with an allowance for new tyres. An employee pocketed the allowance and then spun off the road, killing a pedestrian. The fact that it was their own car and the client had taken all the actions described provided some mitigation. However, the lawyers were left to explain why it was so easy for the employee to lie and run the risk they ran.

In this area, the way to ensure that new systems and procedures are effective is the same, through the analysis, facilitation and user involvement principles that form the core of good BBS.

Summary

When planning a behavioural approach:

- Have a cross-functional team think through all the options.
- Tailor the essentials and consider the desirables.
- Make as systemic, joined-up and holistic a plan as viable, ideally something agreed by operations, SHE, HR and the unions.
- Ensure that no false economies are included by thinking about the politics of the smoke shack. Things that a 'desk jockey' might consider inspirational might land like a lead balloon in the canteen.
- Don't worry about it. If the top-level commitment is genuine, you'll be forgiven!
- Systemically follow it through because embedding is everything.

This will sound like a list of the obvious, but I can't count how many BBS programmes we've reviewed that score badly on one or more of this short list!

7   Person-focused methodologies and human factors

One way to address the fact that many of our accidents are due to people factors is to get the people who work for you to attend something like a fire-walking course. These may look face-valid, but should only be seen as such through the prism of being easy to set up when someone's looking for a magic bullet.

Rather than dismiss such courses out of hand, I'd like to briefly consider how they are supposed to work to engender long-term change psychologically, as this can be enormous fun, hugely empowering and can indeed change your life.

Studies show that boiled-down success in life comes down to two inter-linked things. The first is hard work, which has a huge impact on how much luck you might need (see the Heinrich principle), while the second, related principle is a positive mental attitude, which focuses your behaviours on the process, and not the outcome. For example, studies show it's far better to tell a student that their *hard work* is admirable, as that principle works everywhere and for everything. Telling a student they are *clever* helps their esteem in the short-term, but studies find they can become protective of this mental image, feeling that they don't need to try hard, or even at times deliberately not try-ing hard so that they have an excuse for failure that allows their self-image to remain unaffected.

In *Black Box Thinking*, Matthew Syed relates the story of basketball super-star Shaquille O'Neal. The young player apparently returned from a training camp as a youth, where, for the first time in his life, he didn't stand out as exceptional. Demotivated by this reality check, he moped about for a while and his mother challenged him about his reduced practice. 'I'll do some later', he promised, but his mother replied, 'Remember, for many people, later *never comes*'. This worked. Her words chimed as an eternal truth.

My own 'get it' moment was in a bar in Graz University in southern Austria when, as a layabout, hitchhiking 22-year-old dropout, I suggested to a student friend that I could have gone to university and one chap round the bar table sneered. He didn't quite lean over and patronizingly pat me on the head, but it came close enough. I could have dismissed him as rude, but in a moment of clarity I realized if I didn't do something about it, I would spend the rest of my life having this same conversation with people like him, and ran back to Wales to enrol in an evening class in sociology – the only one with any space left.

More recently, while running a course in Berlin, I talked to Hugh, a delegate who took a year out in the 1970s to lead a convoy of trucks across Europe to Nepal. He agreed that the experience was 'life-changing', but thought it was a nonetheless reasonably uneventful journey, all things considered. Then he added, 'Well, except for that day we were shot at by Turkish MIG fighter planes . . . then there was the day we rescued . . .'.

As a rule, we only have one or two moments of real clarity, and some are unfortunate enough to not have any, but these are nearly always about realizing our potential or making a fundamental change to our life. We 'get it' and then importantly we 'stay got'. This may well be while travelling, at a funeral or after reading an inspirational book. But these moments are few and far between. We watch a film such as Frank Capra's 1946 *It's a Wonderful Life*, starring James Stewart as a small-town person making a huge difference to the lives of others just by being kind and decent. We 'get it' and leave promising to be a better person, but most of us slip back to old habits in a day or two. ABC analysis explains why – just too many short-term temptations!

The point is: we really don't 'stay got' very often. Once or twice in a lifetime, maybe. And even when we do stay got, it's not often about something as specific as safety.

When an inspirational trainer says at the end of a fun course featuring fire-walking, 'Gather around and remember: if you can do this, you can do anything', do you get it? The response will be, 'Hell yeah' and a big group cheer with hugs. It makes for great fun and a great team-bonding exercise, but isn't a foolproof way of improving your organization's safety culture in the long-term. In a group of 20, it's exceptional if as many as five 'stay got', and four of those will head straight to the basketball court, the driving range or the attic room where they were about to give up on the novel they'd been working on.

For a genuine behavioural step change, we need to impact on 50% in the medium- to long-term.

There's valid and merely face-valid, and they can look very similar on a given day – especially if budgets are tight and you need to tick a box for the benefit of HQ.

Awareness-raising case studies

The most moving 'please don't hurt yourself' piece I've even seen was from a South American CEO who opened a safety day with a talk about the most difficult decision he'd ever had to make. One of his workers had been killed some months before, and a situation arose that was passed upwards like a hot potato until it reached his desk. The dead man's desk had finally been reallocated and needed clearing, but they had a problem. His 12-year-old son rang it every day simply to hear his dad's voice so he could pretend he was just in work and would be back later.

In a similar vein, as part of an inspirational talk, a lifeboat volunteer explained the protocol for rescuing families from the sea and how one of the crew is designated the role of keeping children out of the way as they emotionally implore, 'Save my mum', often grabbing at the arms of crew members and impeding the ongoing rescue. 'What happens if you get a big strapping adult out first and their children are still in the sea?' I asked, and was told, 'That's just not viable, so basically you push them back in until we're ready for them'.

Work Safe Victoria in Australia (see worksafe.vic.gov.au) has a DVD that, to a soaring Dido soundtrack, shows a variety of scenes from a Melbourne suburb as people come back from work. It's clever and even amusing in places, but keeps cutting back to a cute and increasingly anxious-looking 10-year-old, and it becomes apparent as the music builds to a climax that his dad *isn't* going to be coming home.

As we reach the end of the clip, half the audience are dabbing at their eyes, but then the dad *does* breeze home safely after all to the exit line: 'The most important reason for being safe at work isn't at work at all'. Exhale and thank the Lord for that. As it's both deeply moving and positive, it fits perfectly with a proactive 'culture creation' approach.

I'll never forget any of these stories, but this isn't BBS; this is awareness-raising, though it does have a place in a holistic approach. Once we have people's full attention, we can do something specific and targeted with them.

Human factors: a more specific and systemic person focus

Realizing that last year's fire-walking course, the previous year's raft-building and the inspirational speaker from the course before that didn't deliver long-term improvement in behaviour, organizations discuss calling in a human factors specialist.

They will ideally tailor their generic model to suit an organization's specific issues, then roll out a fascinating course covering something such as the following list of 'traps', with each error trap coming with a suggested avoidance technique. I'll produce one in full here:

- Norms – avoid bad ones by always maintaining a questioning attitude.
- Complacency – requires a questioning attitude and a pre-job briefing.
- Time pressure – pre-job briefing, questioning attitude and good communication.
- Poor communication – clear communication and a questioning attitude.
- Resource planning – good communication and a questioning attitude.
- Distraction – dynamic risk assessment.
- Interruption – dynamic risk assessment.
- Passivity – communication and a questioning attitude.

- Fatigue – pre-job briefing and communication.
- Stress – communication and a questioning attitude.
- Lack of teamwork – communication and pre- and post-job briefings.
- Lack of technical knowledge – communication, a questioning attitude, pre-job briefing and independent verification.

A good ergonomist would want to boil this down to a list no more than seven points. But what we have here is a systemic consideration of the variety of ways things can go wrong and an excellent basis for a targeted behavioural safety process.

Training employees in this and empowering people to be mindful or to always have a questioning attitude is certainly an excellent start, but how far does it go? As part of a day's course, the issue of passivity will get around half an hour of coverage – just about enough time for the group to agree that the examples given by the trainer are valid and to gather around a flip chart in small groups and come up with a few of their own.

This is still nothing more than a good interactive *briefing and awareness-raising session*. Even the most systemic list from a word-class ergonomist (the above list is from the Atomic Energy Industry) is just edging away from base 1 and maybe pointing at base 2.

It's certainly not embedded, situation-specific *training*, which in this case would perhaps involve *assertion training*. Do you remember the Scott Geller joke about training and education from Chapter 2?

8 A 'don't do that' approach

Following well-designed training in human factors issues, an obvious next step is to design a methodology that seeks to find and address the issues systematically. This is a meaningful and important step forward.

There are various versions, with DuPont's 'STOP' most certainly the best known. This is the top-down behavioural approach often called 'felt leadership', even by organizations who have designed and adapted an in-house version of this approach, which emphasizes a hugely important principle over and above a briefing, no matter how good that briefing might be. This is that safety has to be an ongoing *process* led by line management leading from the front by investing the time to go out into the workplace and engage the workforce in conversations about safety. They coach to enhance discovered learning, and of course always lead by example with the mindset that no accident is inevitable.

There are numerous variations on the exact definition of felt leadership, depending on the consultant or in-house programme leader giving the talk or who wrote the paper/tailored the methodology. At its core is a commitment to turning DuPont's 10 core principles of safety management into reality through day-to-day interactions. These are:

1. All injuries can be prevented.
2. Everyone is responsible for safety.
3. Safety is a condition of employment.
4. Safety needs training.
5. Never stop checking how you're doing.
6. Everyone has the right to challenge anyone – and expect action.
7. There are no minor injuries.
8. Workplace safety is only half the story.
9. Everyone is valuable; we can all learn from each other
10. Never think you can't keep improving.

Unlike the 'if you can walk on hot coals, you can do anything' approach, it's definitely worthy of a BBS badge, and probably the one that most companies use, especially if we add the in-house-designed variations.

Why saying 'don't do that' can often be a good thing

We are clearly moving from '*you* make sure you're safe' to '*we* need to make sure it's safe'. It's an important distinction. The Bradley Curve, devised in a moment of inspiration just before a key meeting, deep inside DuPont by a Vernon Bradley, suggests that organizational culture moves from *dependent* ('I act safely when I'm being watched') through *independent* ('I act safely even when I'm not being watched') to *interdependent* (I am my brother's keeper). It's a conceptual model that resonates as face-valid around the world, but the linear nature of the model can be challenged. In fact, experience suggests that most employees will start at independent but become dependent and disempowered through factors such as learned helplessness where an organization's culture is weak.

It gives us a chance to learn directly from the people undertaking the work, and the inquiry into the Columbia shuttle disaster gives a good example. The chairwoman of the mission management team was asked what she did about dissenting opinions. She replied that, when they heard about them, she took them on board. But when she was asked what she did about dissenting opinions that the team didn't get to hear about and how it set out about going to *find* them, there was an infamous silence.

Being out and about, we also get the chance to actively coach, praise and lead by example. But there's something almost as important that's squarely in the unspoken, subconscious grey area that this book has sought to address. It's because it turns strangers into casual acquaintances, and the culture between acquaintances is much stronger than one between strangers. The civil rights

"BRADLEY CURVE"

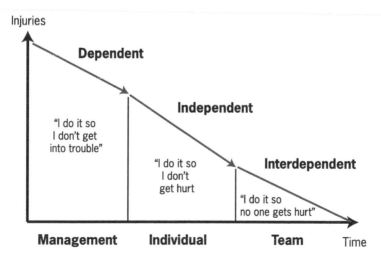

Figure 8.1 Classic Bradley Curve

protestor Rosa Parks is a good example. She wasn't the first person to be arrested in Montgomery for refusing to give up her seat, but she was the first well-known person in town to do so. The 17 others were processed and released, but Rosa was on many committees and made dresses for the wealthy elite, so when she was arrested lots of calls were made and people mobilized.

We respond, at an instinctive physiological level, far more positively to acquaintances then to strangers. Indeed, in some case, we behave far better in front of acquaintances than friends, as we put our best foot forward and are more reluctant to say no to them.

For a BBS programme to work well, and for the benefit of a safety culture, we want an organization made up of acquaintances. Walk-and-talks really help with this and mean that people are far more likely to open up to us when we ask them about realities, or even proactively seek us out. An ever-present questioning attitude is also far more likely to happen when you're with an acquaintance than with a stranger. Similarly, the concept that it's OK to challenge and to be challenged works better too. However, saying that 'challenging and being challenged are valued in this organization' is one thing, but for it to be a day-to-day reality, a lot of groundwork needs to be done. A lot of often self-conscious bridges need to be built so that these behaviours become habit.

Weaknesses

What can go wrong with this walk-and-talk BBS methodology? Or perhaps, where could it go more right? Well, in quite a lot of places.

At its worst, a walk-and-talk methodology can descend close to farce in the paternalistic style it adopts. I once reviewed a training course for a client where a video included as one step of the methodology, 'Bob will now use the technique of listening to Billy'. I'm pretty sure too that the video said this was its '*patented* technique of listening' (™ pending).

A second problem is that often the approach is to reinforce the status quo, also coming from an overly paternalistic position. In another DVD, a manager talking sensibly about workforce empowerment uses the expression 'down there' when referring to the workforce, while someone else reveals with a straight face that 'the workforce may know how your system works even better than you yourself'.

I'd like to walk through the nine-step SUSA approach, as described in the film *Safety Watch (Outtakes 1996)*. Then I'd like to suggest a five-step approach I feel addresses the issues. Finally, I'll cover some contextual problems seen with any sort of walk-and-talk approach. From the US, I'll also consider Geller's seven key behavioural principles to 'applied behavioural science' or 'person-based safety'.

SUSA stands for *Safe and Unsafe Auditing*, and is championed by the consultant John Ormond, formerly of ICI.

I've seen John and colleagues present on this material several times, and I've also undertaken strengths, weaknesses, opportunities and threats (SWOT) analysis of previous behavioural and cultural change programmes based on STOP, SUSA or an in-house version of them.

The nine-step model:

1   Stop and observe people.
2   Put people at their ease.
3   Explain what you're doing and why.
4   Ask about the job: 'What are you doing and what are the stages?'
5   Praise aspects of safe behaviour.
6   Ask, 'What's the worst that could happen and how?'
7   Question 'Why?' of any unsafe behaviour.
8   Ask what corrective action is required.
9   Achieve a commitment to act.

This is clearly a very thorough approach. However, while there's a lot of very good stuff in there, I'll argue that it's rather *too* thorough and a bit top-down. I'll try to justify those observations by addressing the logic and practicality of each point as we walk through.

Geller's seven principles of ABS interlink and overlap rather more perhaps, and so are harder to walk through systemically, but are:

1   Focus on observable behaviour.
2   Look for external factors to understand and improve behaviour.
3   Direct with activators and motivate with consequences.
4   Focus on positive consequences to motivate.
5   Apply the scientific method to improve intervention.
6   Use theory to integrate information, not to limit possibilities
7   Design interventions with consideration of internal feelings and attitudes.

Again, I'll refer to the practicalities of his approach as and when they come up in the SUSA list.

It's worth pointing out here that in point 5, 'the scientific method' is 'define, observe, intervene and test' (DOIT), which is very analogous to BST's BAPP approach.

1 Stop and observe people

This element stresses that observation must be active and will require concentration, hard work and effort, and some dedicated time. The analogy is with 'active listening', which, when done properly, is rather hard work. The famous basketball scene ice-breaking exercise also applies (see www.the invisiblegorilla.com/videos.html for a simple example). This is the scene where delegates are challenged to count passes between intermingling basketball players, some dressed in yellow, some in black. The real question is whether the large gorilla that walks across the scene blows a kiss or beats his chest. The majority of delegates, distracted by the players, will ask, 'What gorilla?'

The overlap with Geller's 'focus on observable behaviour' is obvious, but appreciating that changing attitudes is a very time-consuming affair, Geller also means, 'Don't try and change behaviour via attitudes'. When we are told we have a bad attitude, we will typically respond that we don't', and Freudian concepts such as denial, distortion, rationalization and projection apply. However, on the positive side, 'cognitive dissonance' shows that we don't like our behaviours and attitudes to be out of line, so if we can get people to behave safely, then often the attitude will follow.

Classically, when we persuade a borderline employee to get actively engaged in some aspect of the process that they find rewarding, they announce they have always been fully committed to safety.

Geller's third principle, direct with activators and motivate with consequences, also applies here to an extent, as he's clear that ABC analysis shows that unsafe behaviours are performed for a reason that makes sense to the person at the time. So we have to 'work' that perception.

2 Put people at their ease

Do this by introducing yourself and explaining who you are, what you're doing and why. It's considered vital that you come across as friendly, concerned and constructive. You establish a rapport and that you're there because you care.

This is my first area of concern. This principle can't be faulted, but this is the first hint of *'paternal* parent' in assertion terminology. Done badly, it can come across as a little ominous (as in there's a 'but' coming up here) or even a little patronizing. 'I want you to know I'm here for you' is fine in a Hollywood film but a difficult line to deliver on a North Sea oil rig.

It must be said that the delightful and sincere Ormond *himself* would always get away with it, of course, but the problem is that he doesn't do every one of them. I'd suggest the answer is putting people at their ease by being natural with them, rather than making an effort to do it.

3 Explain what you're doing and why

It's said that the average person can only handle seven items at any one time. And, for many of us, the spread of plus or minus two means we can only manage five or six. Personally, I find myself more and more drawn to the use of triptychs – trios. No list of this sort should ever be longer than seven, and this for me is the first element of repetition that needs to be amalgamated.

It's merely the non-controversial element of point 2. That said, we've reviewed versions where people don't tell the recipient what's happening and why 'to keep them on their toes'. Don't do this, unless you're the CEO, doing an incognito 'back to the floor' exercise that can prove hugely illuminating.

BEFORE HIS INTERPERSONAL SKILLS TRAINING, PAUL'S
ATTEMPTS AT CHALLENGING UNSAFE
BEHAVIOUR DIDN'T ALWAYS WORK OUT

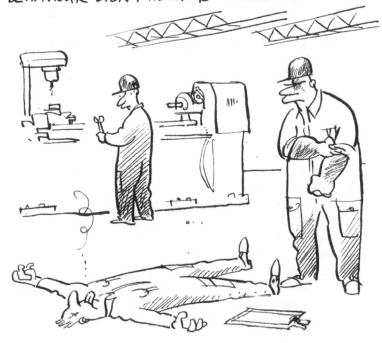

Figure 8.2 The unintended consequence of a badly delivered challenge

4 Ask about the job: 'What are you doing and what are the stages?'

Here, it's stressed that the questions should be open-ended rather than closed. We want the individual to talk in depth and openly, not retreat behind closed answers. For example, asking, 'Are there any safety aspects of this task that concern you?' is likely to get a 'no' from someone wary of your motives or under time pressure. '*What* are the safety implications of doing this task?' is a better question, followed by '*Which* aspects concern you most?' or something along those lines.

This is good stuff, and an excellent way of breaking the ice and starting on some analysis.

5 Praise aspects of safe behaviour

Again, absolutely! However, this is another area where the question 'How skillfully?' is raised, as is the question 'And when?' For example, in the

Safety Watch DVD, Ormond stresses the importance of not being phony, stiff or formal, 'like in the old training films', but then gives the example, 'I noticed you were lifting with a straight back . . . you're not going to be one of those with a bad back'. Again, someone as passionate about safety as John himself will get this right, but it is, I'd argue, uncomfortably close to the 'old training films' John himself warns against that so often go down so badly. Similarly, and to an extent infamously, many upbeat 'way to go Joe' US training films simply don't travel at all well. (Here's a challenge: Read the Australian book *Don't Tell Mum I Work on the Rigs: She Thinks I'm a Piano Player in a Whore House* by the Australian oil worker Paul Carter. The tales he relates are hair-raising, but an excellent example of the daily realities many workers face and the cynical black humour they so often use to get through the day. How careful would you be to get the pitch *exactly* right if Paul and his colleagues were in a safety session you were running?)

The US book *The One Minute Manager* by Ken Blanchard and Spenser Johnson exhorts us to 'catch a person doing something right', and this of course reflects Geller's fourth principle (focus on positive consequences).

Many macho or shy supervisors around the world struggle to use praise comfortably *at all*, so will either avoid it entirely or will try their best but get it wrong. To address this, I'd suggest that whatever process you choose incorporates a praise technique best suited to your local culture.

I'd also suggest that this element *follows* analysis and comes at the end of the session, so that rapport is more likely to have been built, or indeed during the session if it flows naturally. It's actually easier to say, 'That was really interesting. You've given me some real food for thought here, thank you' at the *end* of a discussion than in the middle. So it's easy to imagine a conscientious delegate thinking, 'Right, step 5 . . . praise them now . . . er . . .' and an uncomfortable period following.

6 Ask, 'What's the worst that could happen and how?'

As Ormond says, 'This is a really interesting bit'. This is dynamic risk assessment in action, and also looks to encourage discovered learning, which is the very best form of learning, since thinking of something and articulating it is an *active* process.

On the DVD, Ormond gives an example of a discussion around carrying a container of corrosive material. The observer was concerned that any cracks could lead to the leaking of this corrosive material or that dropping it would lead to fracturing the container and therefore splashing. This was intended as a lead-in to a discussion of the need for suitable PPE and the option of using carrying devices. However, the answer was, 'If I drop it, it may well explode'. So, a discussion that was apparently about PPE and manual handling became a process safety debate.

Clearly, this is just the very heart of a good discussion.

7 Question 'Why?' of any unsafe behaviour

As a passionate believer in the Just Culture perspective, I'd consider this element utterly vital and non-controversial – though it shouldn't be just one thing towards the end of a list of *nine*.

Geller is hugely systematic here, and this is his second principle: 'look for external factors'. Specifically, he suggests a number of questions a facilitator can ask, including:

- Can the task be simplified to make it more user-friendly? He also suggests asking if unsafe behaviour is rewarded, which, referring back to ABC analysis (speed and comfort are rewarding in themselves), is simply another way of asking the same question.
- Are there basic barriers to safety, such as an individual being unaware of how to work safely, not having the right physical or psychological profile, or the relevant equipment not being available?
- Is safe behaviour punished (including peer-teasing as well as speed issues)?
- Is the law of unintended consequences applying, because, for example, bonuses are driving under-reporting?
- If it's a critical skill that might well drift over time, do we follow it up? Most obviously, this is applicable to emergency response dummy runs.

I've amalgamated and paraphrased a really extensive list of highly useful questions, but nowhere in there will you find anything *directly* relating to leader member exchange or culture, or the ways these interactions directly determine behaviour and perception. This is key, as once the stage of diminishing returns has been reached in terms of the basics of competence and compliance, which happens at most companies, then subtle cultural cues are about half of what's left.

The crux of this for me is this direct quote from the Geller overview article in *The Handbook of Occupational Safety and Workplace Health* from 2015:

> A systematic behavior analysis of risky work practices can pinpoint many determinants of such behavior, including inadequate management systems or supervisor behaviors that promote or inadvertently encourage at risk work.

It's a simple mindset issue, but becomes incredibly important once we consider how training cascades and reverts to the status quo in the middle of a busy shift. However, I suggest substituting the '*can*' in the above sentence with '*will typically*'. If we see this determinant as a probability, rather than a *possibility*, and look for reasons to actively rule it out, then our analysis will be more accurate and the resulting actions more effectively targeted.

Such tinkering might provoke horror that I am daring to mildly criticize the man who invented the term to describe this concept and has decades of successful consultancy behind him, or question the Behaviour-Based Accident Prevention Process (BAPP), which has saved thousands of lives around the world and tens of thousands of injuries. But I'm not suggesting a heretical revolution; it's a simple but vital nudge-inspired *evolution*.

I'm simply saying that Krause, Geller, Daniels, *et al.* should, by now, have absorbed the thinking of Dekker, Reason and Hopkins and fine-tuned their BBS methodologies. In his excellent BBS overview of 2015, from which the above quote comes, Geller references key papers by luminaries in the field of behaviourism or behavioural science, such as Festinger, Zohar, Krause, Daniels, McSween, Skinner and Deming (it's a very thorough article), but makes no mention of Just Culture or the hugely influential works on influencing skills by Thaller, Sunstein and Cialdini. And as evidence of the validity of the charge that this American model is all a bit insular and self-referencing, it's worth pointing out that his overview article references *himself* 29 times. Similarly, in Tom Krause's excellent *Leading with Safety*, Krause gives himself 16 references, while Kahneman gets only one, and there are none for Reason, Dekker or Hopkins.

My issue is that even the best person-centred approach is, by definition, still *person*-centred. It's almost impossible to find a situation where there is nothing that can be *learned* and where empathy and proactive analysis isn't appropriate, so unless we fluke it, the efficacy of our response is limited by the quality of our understanding. *Starting with learning* is also often really helpful from a methodological view, as many workers *can't* be observed.

It should not be learning as a part of a classic observation and feedback approach, as Geller suggests, but observation (if used) as part of an analysis and learning-based approach that proactively and directly enhances the environment. All methodologies should flow from this.

At the end of his article, Geller raises several challenges for BBS going forward, including:

- What do we do for sustainability over and above the observation and feedback process?
- How can we develop a 'brother's keeper' or interdependence culture, so that peer-to-peer feedback is supportive and corrective?
- How does the active involvement of management impact on a BBS process?

A European/Australian view is already addressing these issues. In 'B is for BBS' (March 2016 *IOSH* magazine), Bridget Leathley demonstrates a welcome focus on analysis, not coaching. She gives the example that if people are slipping on a wet floor, one should not just ask people to walk carefully. The approach should be to fix any leak and, if that's not possible, limit the number of people who walk on it and issue non-slip footwear. The top of the slips and trips hierarchy is change the flooring. This is 'several whys', or really excellent 'hazard elimination', which, as Leathley rightly says, 'BBS is no substitute for.'

Even this article stops short of mentioning a holistic approach including culture and leadership. In response to objective analysis-based recommendation, the question 'You're saying we need to change the flooring?' can be asked in a variety of voice tones. Some may require an exclamation mark. And some may *really* need an exclamation mark! (like that).

To directly address Geller's challenges:

- What do we do for sustainability over and above the observation and feedback process? *(A learning-based approach doesn't even have observation as the core methodology.)*
- How can we develop a 'brother's keeper' (interdependence) culture, so that peer-to peer feedback is supportive and corrective? *(By building a strong culture where challenging and being challenged, if required, is stress-free. That's primarily a cultural issue, where empathy and mutual respect is key, so start with a listening and learning methodology based on that.)*
- How does the active involvement of management impact on a BBS process? *(They listen, they facilitate and they praise BBS work. Sometimes they coach. Sometimes they need to challenge, but they always play **the** central role in a holistic set of methodologies that is 'cultural safety'.)*

In short, we shouldn't see BBS methodologies as a stand-alone, but a key element of a holistic approach to cultural excellence and cultural safety. Process and personal safety are just overlapping subsets, as are health and well-being. The explicitly BBS element, as most know it, isn't primarily peers challenging peers about unsafe behaviour; it is peers *conversing* with peers about the causes of and solutions to risk issues.

8 Ask what corrective action is required

Coaching and discovered learning skills are central to this element, as getting an individual to articulate what needs to be done is active for them. There is a loop back here to analysis of course and the DVD stresses that the observer might get an answer they weren't expecting, in particular that they might well get a *better* answer than they themselves could have come up with. Again, I'd like to suggest that the underlying tone is one of paternal expert pleasantly surprised by workers' thoughts and knowledge.

That underlying tone is everything, so it's vital to always work from the *assumption* that the person you are talking to is thoughtful and more knowledgeable than you can ever hope to be about the task in hand, unless they prove conclusively otherwise.

Specifically, it is suggested in the DVD that 'a training need might be identified'. This doffs a cap at Just Culture and blameless error, but the wording is key and is the nub of my concern about the approach, because a training need is a *person*-focused response. Coming at this from a Just Culture perspective, a training need *might* well be identified, but it's just as likely to be in *management* and shouldn't be the first thing to jump to mind. Specifically, needing to address the way the task is set up and resourced is, in most cases, a statistically more likely answer.

We're in a minefield of nuances here, of course. The distinction I've just made may sound pedantic to many companies and managers, but *not* if you are genuinely coming at this discussion with Dekker's 'new view' or Conklin's 'pre-accident investigation' in mind.

9 Achieve a commitment to act

This very explicitly means *from the person being observed*. Of course, that's now the obvious closeout to a conversation of this type. It's what we were building to all along, and this is really the clinching piece of evidence here as to why I think these approaches are too paternal, because from a paternal perspective this makes total sense. People are acting unsafely and they need to commit to stopping that, but this is squarely in 'we need to talk about your behaviour' territory.

Sometimes this will be appropriate, but if 90% of the causes of unsafe behaviour are *environmental*, wouldn't simple logic dictate that 90% of these closeout commitments to act should come from the *observer*?

Trusted leaders 'eat last', and eliciting promises from workers not to repeat an unsafe act is the thing they should do last, if at all.

In summary, SUSA-style methodologies continue to be used successfully by a variety of organizations all around the world. Ormond and the other users will, I imagine, stress that, of course, there is training given to delegates to support the approach, which addresses many of the points I've made. They may also have made changes to the approach, having read some Dekker.

I'd argue that the paternal parent mindset isn't where a world-class mindset sits. It needs to be adult-to-adult *always*, as it minimizes the chance of nouns turning into verbs.

To explain: when we undertake surveys, one of the cultural clues we look for is *how* a programme is referred to.

'Let's do a SUSA' (i.e. together) is fine.

'I'm going to do a SUSA' is OK-ish.

'I'm going to SUSA you' is not.

Once that later perception has taken hold, then its efficacy as a methodology is inevitably limited. No one will give it a fair go, if nothing else. It's exactly like the cultural commentators who say you can always tell when morale is low in an organization when employees stop saying 'we' and start saying 'them', as in, '*They* need to sort this out'.

It's worth remembering that the vast majority of these audits are undertaken *months*, if not years, after the initial training course, and the more opportunity there is for the wrong tone to be struck or the wrong emphasis given, the more often it will happen. In the heat of battle, people will nearly always boil down a list of nine to a triptych of three and focus on the elements they're most comfortable with. If this is an organization with a pathological compliance focus generally, then benefit will still accrue, but we're in trouble in terms of cultural excellence. If, in addition, the front-line managers have had limited or no soft skills training, that can be *really* asking for trouble. There are plenty of anecdotal examples showing that this is exactly what can result.

I'd like to instead suggest a five-stage model, as detailed in an earlier book, *Talking Safety*.

Summary of recommended 'walk-and-talk' five-stage model

It's worth going back to basics and recalling why we should devote valuable organizational time to undertake a walk-and-talk at all. It is never to try to catch someone out. Instead, it is to:

- physically scan issues such as housekeeping, while out and about;
- learn something about the organization and the people who work there through the eyes of those people, in particular to understand the unspoken but vital *nuances*;
- understand why things have gone wrong or, if nothing wrong is seen, what people can be tempted to do;
- model the behaviours and mindset we want the organization to be built on;
- coach, empower, facilitate and even inspire your colleagues to discovered learning and embedded behaviours; and
- establish rapport, thus making more frequent and better-quality communications about safety more likely in the future.

Occasionally, it is also to:

- insist on an improvement in existing standards of behaviour and approach.

That's a list up for debate and which I've tried to justify. The following approach is designed to more directly map onto these aims.

It's *quality*, not *quantity*, that we're after. We don't have to stay out and about for a set amount of time. The final chapter gives some practical 360-degree-style checklist questions that allow you to check the quality.

1 Introduce yourself and set the tone

You're interested in them and their work, and not trying to impress them with your knowledge, so you'll ask questions and listen to the answers. You might ask about their home life, the task they're undertaking and about process, as well as personal safety issues. You should try to draw them out with a 'what if?' question that shows curiosity, commitment and 'mindfulness' – not an attempt to catch them out. The assumption is that they are intelligent, committed and knowledgeable, until they prove conclusively otherwise.

There's a head of safety of a specialist construction company who, 9 times out of 10, *only* does this during her walk-and-talk. It's proving highly successful, as it covers most of the points in the list above with an explicit aim at learning generally and rapport-building. She finds that when she has to address an issue more directly, her colleagues couldn't be more accommodating.

2 Analysis

If you have seen anything worrying, ask why, but ask it *curiously*, knowing that 90% of the time you'll get something interesting back that's about the organization and environment, not about the individual. If there's an individual element, then minimizing defensiveness will help.

You can proactively start this discussion, even if you've seen nothing, by asking if there's anything slow, uncomfortable or inconvenient about doing this job safely. People will nearly always have something to say here and, if they trust you, they'll tell you. The conversation never has to move from the hypothetical and anonymous, so it's just as useful with peripatetic workers. The learning, however, *isn't* hypothetical.

One of the biggest problems we see with systems such as safety contact is that analysis lacks depth. We often get asked how it is that things aren't getting any better, despite the fact that they've put straight lots of things that have been highlighted over the past year. The answer is that often auditors will list any number of problems but simply generate what's known as a 'crap list' of items that will recur.

Reason uses a mosquito analogy. He suggests that if you have a problem with mosquitoes, then a short-term solution is to buy nets, repellent and swatters, but a better solution is to find the swamp they come from and *drain it at source.*

One of the specific causes of these 'crap lists' is that people are often wary of approaching someone they don't know, especially if they're uncertain of the technicalities of the job. They therefore avoid talking to them at all, and just pick on something visible and easy such as housekeeping, then pop an action point down around that. To an extent, the VIP visit to the Macondo site the day before the explosion was accused of this. A hazard may well be removed as a consequence, and that's always a good thing, but it's not necessarily the optimal use of time.

If you cover the following questions thoroughly, then you'll be bound to have a good discussion that may well generate some self-analysis in the person you're talking to.

Those are:

- What does this job involve?
- What can go wrong? (Include *process* safety issues.)
- What might happen if it did?
- How do we make sure that doesn't happen?

And of course . . .

- Is there anything slow, uncomfortable or inconvenient about that?

Typically, as well as noticing the immediate risk once you've used your Five Whys analysis as above, you may well find yourself considering such points as:

- risk assessments;
- barriers;
- signage;
- supervision;
- suitability of PPE;
- training;
- inductions;
- selection and monitoring of contractors; and
- behaviours that are typical and not remarked on.

Any of these issues worked through *systematically* and analytically and turned into an action plan is a long way from a basic hazard spot. But doing this systematically will nearly always require an in-depth conversation with the person doing the job. And that's where a dedicated open-minded safety contact comes in.

Two elephants in the room

An excellent 'walk-and-talk' looking for personal safety issues should also look for the two thumping great elephants in the room: process safety and health. Hopkins says this well:

> The behavioral approach is just as applicable to process safety as it is to personnel safety and auditing and monitoring activities should cover both. One of the criticisms leveled at behavioral safety generally is that it ignores process safety. It is vital that behavioral safety programs face this challenge.

Absolutely! And when we consider the numbers, everything that applies to process safety applies 100-fold to health issues. On 'walk-and-talks', we should, of course, talk about obvious risks such as falling down the stairs, but we should also talk about unlikely but catastrophic risks and delayed but personally catastrophic risks relating to long-term health. Awareness of mental health issues is increasing worldwide year by year, so, though it may have been asked above already, 'How are you?' is always worth asking.

3 Coaching

You're already fully in coaching mode and modelling the mindset we want. If there is some specific learning you want to actively impart, however, you need to use questions to maximize discovered learning. More often, you'll just want to be using coaching techniques to lead them through a chain of thought. Following the three golden rules, as illustrated by the feedback fish, means you can't go far wrong: a slightly more detailed discussion about the feedback fish, the use of praise and coaching excellence follows. But in summary:

- You ask questions (then 'rate yourself 1 to 10' perhaps).
- They say it first, proving they knew it, and therefore maximizing ownership of it.
- You maximize the praise opportunities that flow from this.

4 Promises

If you've done the first three properly, then any promises required will be likely to have been made *internally* already, which is vital as this means they are far more likely to be *kept* when you're not around. There are times, however, when we need a promise to be made genuinely because of a clear and present risk that can't be designed out in the near future or maybe can't be designed out at all because of the cost.

I once worked on an oil platform where using the hand-over-hand climbing technique, unencumbered by trying to carry materials, was key on several vertical ladders as feet often slipped on the rungs. This was because the rungs had been designed for average-sized feet. That might seem perfectly reasonable, but it meant that anyone with large feet hadn't the ideal clearance, and toes often snagged. We looked into replacing the ladders, but they were an integral part of the initial platform design. So, as well as a behavioural red flag, it was one for the designers to keep in mind next time around.

Organizations are often chock-full of such problems. When Piper Alpha was upgraded to cope with gas, for example, there was a firewall added, as gas is flammable. But it wasn't blast-proof, and gas fires tend to follow gas explosions. When organizations can get this sort of thing wrong, built-in behavioural issues will abound.

A top tip from influencing skills

Cialdini *et al.* have many nudge-influenced tips for getting people to keep promises. Perhaps the most relevant for this part of a safety conversation is the use of the 'I' word. People who look you in the eye and say 'I will' are about five times less likely to break that promise than people who mumble at their feet.

If you ask someone to look after something important for you and they mumble, 'Yeah, yeah, sure', without catching your eye, you'd be a fool trust them. By looking them square in the eye and asking, 'Will you, please?' you maximize the chance of them looking back and answering, 'Yes I will'. It's largely subconscious, and they may well be unaware of those fingers they had crossed behind their back being uncrossed.

5 Close out and follow up

Thank people sincerely for their time and insight. Turn anything that needs doing into a SMART goal and then follow up and close out – or delegate a follow-up to ensure it was closed out. In addition to specific benefits, this also shows our genuine commitment.

Just Culture shows that around 9 times out of 10, the person who needs to take an action away from the encounter is the one with the 'clipboard'. We know that capital projects can be frustrating and time-consuming to set up, and that we can all get so focused on the day-to-day realities that we're tempted to put long-term issues on the back burner. Basically, in the short-term, it's a relief.

It's vital that we don't file it in the back of the filing cabinet, but actually stick to the SMART timetable, and the person involved is returned to and updated on progress. If someone else is asked to talk to them, then don't cross it off the to-do list as 'delegated' until it's checked that they actually did.

Summary of the five-step model

Executed well, a good 'walk and talk' will deliver savings through:

- less time and effort spent enforcing rules and regulations that are impractical or contradictory;
- less admonishment of employees who are honestly trying their best and resent being 'unfairly told off', with a consequent impact on discretionary effort and other 'psychological contract' issues; and
- a reduction in 'crap lists', which, while diligently circulated and rectified, simply recur time after time.

I've tried to make this version shorter and more analysis-focused for two main reasons. One is because this models Just Culture and the 'new view' of error, and most accurately models what's actually going on and why. Second, because it minimizes the chance of the methodology skewing to something less positive down the line.

If you're not going to do anything directly with the workforce as part of the BBS strategy, then I'd strongly suggest that this is the one systemic process you do install.

The key is to use the learning generated to provide management with suitable training in associated generic skills, and embed and support them properly by following up with a basic 360-degree approach that checks for quality as well as quantity and supports strugglers with some coaching.

If you do this, I guarantee that, at the very least, the number of risky behaviours will absolutely plummet.

A related practical problem: a lack of planning

If you fail to plan, you plan to fail, as the saying goes. So what planning is required of a 'walk–and–talk'?

First, we should check any 'walk–and–talk' databases or review previous safety contacts, and consider:

- Who went on–site last and what did they target?
- What did they find?
- What actions resulted? And how are things progressing?

Also, a basic:

- Consideration of which jobs are being undertaken and when . . .

This will help ensure you don't turn up looking to target the same things as the last person. For example, you might note that no one has targeted working at height for a while so you could look to target that.

You could, of course, find yourself waiting forever for it to be totally convenient to undertake a safety contact audit, so don't be too timid. However, please do show some discretion. If it's obvious that the people you need to talk to are *absolutely* flat-out busy, or if interrupting them could actually be dangerous, then give them some space and look at something else for a while. While you must make it clear you're not going to be fobbed off and leave, please *do* empathize and put yourself in their shoes. Simply ask yourself what would be reasonable if they were making an effort.

A little empathy and intelligence is all that's required, and that's also true of the next chapter on generic skills.

9 Generic skills

This chapter describes some skills that should always be included in training a holistic BBS approach. This applies to managers and supervisors, and may more usually come under the banner of 'safety leadership', but should also cover any front-line volunteers because the way they conduct themselves will resonate too. There are also some techniques that are often included, or are increasingly being included, but which perhaps shouldn't be.

Such generic skills include soft skills, analysis techniques and influencing skills. Let's start with nudge theory, which can be argued to include many influencing and soft skills.

'Nudge theory' or 'behavioural economics'

Nudge theory, as popularized by Richard Thaler and Cass Sunstein, can be defined as making a change to the environment that is clever, cheap, based on an understanding of psychology and physiology, and validated. The most famous nudge is the painted fly on the toilet in Amsterdam Airport Schiphol, which men can't help but point at, with a reduction in splashing of up to 80% leading to an associated improvement in cleaning costs and the environmental impact of cleaning materials.

Crucially, this idea came from the man tasked with keeping the toilets clean. This is not coincidental.

It has been suggested that nudge is just manipulation – clever ideas for getting you to do what the organization wants without you realizing that's what they did it. Well yes, but *flattery* achieves much the same objective.

It's also suggested that nudge theory has been around forever, and indeed it has. The famous 'Hawthorne effect' study was originally about painting factory walls different colours to get the employees to work harder. It found that if you make a change, it gives a boost, and that it didn't much matter whether the wall was painted red, green or yellow. The crucial factor was that it was given a new colour. That said, the colour of walls *can* be important. The bestseller *Drunk Tank Pink* by Adam Alter, for example, shows that using different colours can increase and decrease aggression levels.

Regardless, anyone who ever got a tin of paint out to make it crystal clear where something, or someone, goes or doesn't go was using 'nudge'. If it really *doesn't want to go there*, then best use *red* of course. Making a change to the environment that is clever, cheap, based on science and an understanding of psychology and physiology, and validated shouldn't be controversial at all when applied to safety, so an increase in the use of behavioural economics should be a good thing in all organizations.

For example, consider an old-fashioned BBS team trained in ABC analysis and how to use an *impact* matrix. Trying to fill up the high–impact, low–cost box with clever ideas about how to make the safe way the convenient way is clearly underpinned by a nudge mindset. Leader member interactions and the shadow they throw is also a fruitful area. It's about systemically ensuring we stop asking, 'Why did you switch off?' and substitute the question, 'Is everything that caused you to switch off now under control?' because the former says, 'You had better have a good reason for that' and the latter communicates, 'Of course you did or you wouldn't have done it . . . what happened?' That's impactful but cheap, so arguably a nudge. Changing 'safely but by Friday' to 'by Friday but safely' is also nudge, because the meaning of the communication is in the words following the 'but'.

A Plymouth University study led by Liz Hellier shows that labels about hazards need to be big and bold, rather than discreet in size. They also need to contain *clear instruction that's personalized*, not mere advice.

Therefore, to ensure a required behaviour, labels need to say, 'You need to do X and Y and must never do Z' on the front in bold lettering under a large hazard sign. A discreet sign on the back with a note advising, 'This is highly toxic so there is a risk of . . .' just doesn't cut it. It's not about basic compliance with regulations, but the efficacy of the message, and we can often massively increase efficacy for very little cost.

Similarly, the same study showed that a safety briefing is as much about where and how it is delivered as it is about content. It's about a smartly dressed person, in a professional environment, delivering a crisp talk backed up with good-quality materials.

This really isn't rocket science, and shouldn't need to be proved by university research. Here's a challenge. Put a team together looking at the effectiveness and impact of warning signs and talks. Even in the best organizations, you'll find some really obvious opportunities. In an average or poor organization, you could be there a while.

In both circumstances, I'd argue this is really good BBS. I'd also like to consider handwashing, a really simple behaviour whose absence costs billions of dollars and millions of lives annually but still needs clever nudging.

Advertising agency Ogilvy & Mather was tasked with getting South American meat workers to wash their hands thoroughly because contamination rates were causing millions of pounds worth of products to be rejected upstream. Its solution was to stamp hands on entry to the factory with a dye that only really thorough washing could get off, and huge savings ensued.

Here, we can quickly cross-reference hospitals around the world and the avoidable secondary infection rates that kill millions every year. In my experience, the health 'industry' is overly defensive and not good at learning or implementing best practice. It doesn't learn readily from the mistakes or innovations of others, and not even always from its own errors. This is one of the biggest HSE challenges of our generation. The contrast with the mindset and culture of the aviation industry is examined in detail in Syed's book *Black Box Thinking*.

It's tempting to suggest that every organization needs a 'nudge' unit looking specifically at safety and health issues. That's a bit redundant, though, as many already have, though some look more at production-based issues and others have different names. However, a BBS team well trained in ABC (or temptation) analysis and impact-matrix use is most definitely a 'nudge' unit.

'Followership'

In 1964, a New York woman, Kitty Genovese, was murdered outside a block of flats in which she lived. She was attacked twice. The first time, dozens of people heard the attack and opened windows to see what was happening, which drove the assailant away. It was reported that no one called the police, however, so when he returned to gawp at the crime scene, she still lay injured where he'd left her, and he resumed the assault. Later, there was controversy when it was claimed a call *was* made, but at least this horrible incident inspired some groundbreaking research into the bystander effect.

Experiments were set up to see how easy it is to 'say something first'. The actual experiment was harder than the simple example (pulled from Wikipedia) below. However, the study found that if you're the unknowing subject, last but one in a long line of stooges who lie and say that B matches the control, then most people will deny the evidence of their own eyes and agree that B is the match. However, if just one person is allowed to break ranks and say that C is the match, then the majority of subjects will say, 'I don't know what the rest of you are seeing, but I agree with X – I think it's C'. It illustrates how reluctant people are to speak up (as on the night of the murder), but also how just one person can make a big difference to the behaviour of others around them.

This is especially powerful if that person is a leader of some description, but they don't have to be. The whole field of followership is gaining increasing attention, especially the vital importance of the person who proves to be the 'first follower'. This is the person first to say, 'That's a good idea, and I'm going to follow them/copy that idea' (see the TED talk by Derek Sivers at www.ted.com/talks/derek_sivers_how_to_start_a_movement?language=en).

The psychology is the same whether we are seeking to reduce passive bystanding or encourage speaking up or first following. It's about empowering people to do or say something when previously they wouldn't have, and then reinforcing these behaviours so that they do them again and they become habit.

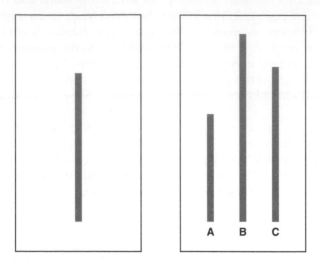

Figure 9.1 The Classic Asch conformity research example

Feedback and coaching

It's important not to confuse delegation with *abdication*. Empowerment is largely based on choice and autonomy, but that's not just allowing people to 'get on with it'. Guidance, coaching or even one-to-one mentoring will also be required as part of a transformational leadership approach. Giving good feedback and even active coaching is central to doing this well.

BST's Behaviour-Based Accident Prevention Process (BAPP) approach has feedback as one of the four cornerstones of its BBS approach, and Dominic Cooper of B-Safe is very strong on this element. In short, feedback is essential to a behavioural approach, or any attempt to improve anything for that matter.

Safety feedback isn't just stage 3 in a structured BBS approach.

Imagine trying to learn to play golf, but blindfolded with no feedback as to where your ball had gone. You'd never improve. Similarly, we all have the accents we have because of feedback. We want to please our parents, so we try to copy what they say, but as we learn they reinforce the sound of key words in their own image. We could teach our children to speak like the Queen of England, but we don't. They speak like us.

Feedback is a subtle thing. It isn't just marching up to someone and saying, 'Well done!' We're constantly receiving feedback; we're not even aware of just picking up an accent. So a supervisor praising us for safe behaviour is a good thing, but it may not be effective if a different supervisor who is more important to us later contradicts that message by saying, 'We all heard Greg before and I'm not going to contradict him. Safety *is* of course the number one priority, but . . .'). The first message will be undermined.

Basic feedback

When someone is observed acting safely, then any praise is a soon, certain and positive reward when delivered from a credible source, and will help reinforce the behaviour. The more of this, the better, and books such as Blanchard's *The One Minute Manager* can help. As above, a key principle in the book is to catch a person doing something right. This is particularly important when a key behaviour has been targeted as suboptimal and in need of improvement. It also holds true regardless of whether it's a behaviour that the workforce could easily have undertaken but aren't doing, such as an enabled one or one that's difficult to do.

This must be part of a damage-limitation approach, while we work out how to make it easy to do.

Regardless, where a behaviour has been recently enabled (perhaps providing handrails where previously there were none), we'll still want to reinforce the holding of them to ensure it embeds and becomes 'what we do around here'.

There's a famous old BBS exercise in which a volunteer is blindfolded and tasked to throw a handful of marker pens or spoons into a bucket from 10 feet away. In the first run, they get no feedback whatsoever; in the second, they receive only negative feedback; and in the third, all the feedback is positive. They typically do badly in the first run, worse in the second and may even refuse to continue if jeered with enough gusto. But they perform better in the third.

Praise is 20 times more effective than criticism in changing behaviour, and catching someone doing something right is a 'soon, certain and positive' pay-off. On the third run, a thrower will instantly improve and will typically hit the bucket in 6 to 10 throws. However, this is still, of course, entirely person-focused, and I've added a fourth iteration here that demonstrates this.

Told that the rules remain in place and that the person throws the pens one at a time, blindfolded and from 10 feet, but that everything else is open to a design or teamwork solution, we soon have funnels and catchers and coaches suggesting a lobbed throw to help the catcher.

This is 100% successful because, while praise may be 20 times better than criticism, it's no substitute for designed facilitation.

Negative feedback

By far the biggest issue with negative feedback is, of course, in many organizations, the utter *lack of it* ('blind eye' syndrome). Because what we fail to challenge, we effectively condone.

'It's OK to be challenged and it's OK to challenge' is an expression often heard in an organization desiring a strong culture, and must be a key aim of any organization seeking excellence. Training people in these skills is the easy part. Creating an environment in which they are used readily is the hard bit.

Specifically, when giving negative feedback, it's vital to follow some key rules, otherwise the impact will be the opposite of that intended. They won't be thinking of the behaviour at hand and any associated risk. They'll be thinking of you, and not in a nice way. If they can, they'll let you know on the spot, usually through their voice tone and body language, but sometimes more directly. If not, they'll just reduce the amount of discretionary effort. Often it'll be both.

The golden rules of giving negative feedback are:

- never personalize;
- never generalize; and
- never berate someone in front of others for extra impact.

A loud 'You're always doing this, you ****' is a funny line to put in a 'Don't do it this way' training video, but *only* there. We rarely do anything 'always', and if you call me that, the only thing I'll be thinking about is its inappropriateness. If you do it in front of my peers, they may laugh, especially if it's frequently true. But I'll spend the rest of the day fantasizing about having you killed. If I'm popular, the colleagues won't laugh. They'll be mortified. Look up 'workplace bullying' in any HR policy. Being criticized in front of colleagues will be high on the list.

Here's an example that has stuck with me over the years, concerning a man who recently died. His name was Dave Fanning of Chep UK, and he was an excellent leader: fair, resolute, consistent, thoughtful, clear in his communications – everything a leader should be. A former rugby league player, he was a key figure in a project that saw accident rates cut to a tenth of previous levels nationwide in 18 months.

One of the things Dave knew how to do was to give feedback for maximum impact *and* minimum unintended consequence. The incident I remember was at a residential training event where one of the employer's trainees was rude to a waitress. It was nothing too serious, but was out of order nonetheless. Dave saw this but said nothing, waited a minute or two, then casually asked the young chap if he could have a quick word about something that had just occurred to him. Unconcerned, the young man followed him out of the room, but when he returned five minutes later he looked shaken and white. Before he left the room, he gave a sincere apology to the waitress.

Normally, tactfully taking someone to the side and sticking objectively to the facts at hand is all that's required. That's exactly what Dave did. He didn't personalize, generalize or raise his voice. But this didn't stop him from articulating his observations very clearly.

In doing so, he'll have done that young chap a service. And that's the point. Negative feedback is sometimes required. However, doing it well is essential. Many an individual avoids the difficulties here by rarely doing it all, and then, like a backfiring motorbike, charging in unadvisedly all guns blazing.

Remember, we are seeking to build a culture of trust and openness conversation-by-conversation.

Advanced feedback

Communications guru Marshall Goldsmith encourages the use of the 'feed forward' technique (see www.marshallgoldsmithfeedforward.com for a free four-minute video). It's simple, and any organization that can use it regularly won't be going far wrong. The idea is that improvement ideas are sought and articulated in a positive way, so to pick up on the above example, don't say, 'You shouldn't shout at him in front of his peers, it'll backfire'.

Instead, he suggests saying, 'He got the message OK, but I'd like to suggest you'd have greater impact in the long-term if you took him to one side to give him that feedback. I worry that he's not thinking about the feedback; he's just thinking about you, and not in a good way'.

The trick is that the person getting the feedback is obliged to do one thing, and one thing only, which is to *treat it like a present*. So we first say, 'Thank you', and then either (a) pop it in a drawer and drop it off at a charity shop later; or (b) use it. Just Culture shows us that it's nearly always the situation, not the person, so we need be good at generating and using ideas as to how to improve the situation.

Clearly this does that. Goldman would be great at leading a BBS team.

Active listening

You'd think that the skill of listening wouldn't take long to master, and it's true that the component parts of an active listening technique are not difficult to grasp. It's using them in action that's tiring and difficult. The component parts are:

- **Pay full attention**

This is not just turning off your phone off, not looking over their shoulder and not cutting them off rudely. Nor is it simply waiting for them to finish speaking so that you can say your thing. It's also about actively listening to what they are saying by watching their body language, remembering that 85% of the communication is in the tone and body language.

- **Paraphrase back what they have said**

Confirm you listened by repeating it back in slightly different language, showing you have *processed* it rather than merely parroting it. And also paraphrase back the meaning you got from it, if there's anything in the 85% that jars.

This is key. If they are saying something but not sounding as if they genuinely meant it, then this is the time to clarify. This doesn't have to be confrontational. Something like, 'John, I'm getting the impression that you have concerns about X and Y . . . could you clarify that?' suffices.

- **Cut the boxing ring down with a 'yes/no' in the face of evasion**

If you feel you're being fed a mixed message *deliberately*, perhaps to pass the problem onto you, then 'yes/no' is your friend. Saying, 'Safely but by Friday' suggests 'by Friday', so a way of clarifying that would be to challenge by asserting, 'I can do it safely and I can do it by Friday, but we both know that I may not be able to do both. What I'm hearing is that, given the choice, you want this out by Friday come what may?' It's likely that our supervisor will bluster, 'Er . . . I didn't say that'. Then, to drive home the point, you will need to ask, 'So, to clarify, if I need to delay until the weekend to ensure no corners are cut, is that OK?'

You may well get an, 'I didn't say that either!' but they are in a situation now where they have to either say one or the other, or clearly refuse to say either. In any inquiry following something going wrong, the initial 'get-out' that they were trying to set up, consciously or otherwise ('I explicitly said do it safely . . . I'm not sure what the problem is'), is now removed. It will be clear to all now that they didn't say anything explicit and tried to fudge it.

It's impossible to overstate the power of listening to someone in an adult-to-adult fashion of mutual respect, then being able to return a week later to say, 'We discussed that idea you came up with last week, agreed it was indeed high-impact and low-cost, and have commissioned it. I just wanted to pop back and say thank you'.

For example, have you ever been stopped in the street by someone with a clipboard who you tried to get past but failed? Did you find yourself five minutes later saying, 'And another thing . . . write this down too' to a person who clearly got what they needed minutes ago? Everyone loves the chance to articulate their thoughts.

Assertion and difficult customers

Being able to give negative feedback well and to challenge mixed messages are key skills of assertion. Assertion is not asserting yourself; it's insisting that your rights be respected without impacting on those of others. An assertive 'argument' might go something like this:

> 'With respect boss, I think X decision is wrong. What about Y factor?'

> 'That's a good point, and actually considering factor Y did indeed give me pause for thought. However, on balance, I still think we should do X, and I get the casting vote.'

> 'OK, I'll try not to say "I told you so" if you're wrong. But that's not a promise.'

The key aspects are mutual respect and that the boss still gets to be the boss. This is an *I'm OK, You're OK* interaction from the classic book of that name.

Of course, mutual respect might be thin on the ground. In this case, techniques such as 'broken record' and 'paraphrasing the message' can be used to show you've listened and understood, without agreeing with it.

Here's a real safety-related example of a very heated exchange I saw using both:

> 'You're just wrong. If we cut down to single manning, then there's no one to cover and raise the alarm if something goes wrong. These phones that raise the alarm if you don't move for a couple of minutes are no substitute. If you're not moving because you've had a heart attack or been stabbed, you want the right help to be on the effing way instantly, not some general "Oh something might be wrong, we'd better investigate" 20 minutes later. It's a disgrace, and you know it.'

> 'I agree there are enhanced risks to the workforce under the new way, but the situation was simple and agreed with all stakeholders. It was: "make significant cost savings, utilizing the very best technology available, or risk being closed entirely".'

> 'That's bull and you know it.'

> 'You've made it clear you're not happy, but this is, as you know, simply the best outcome of those available.'

> 'I say it's an effing disgrace!'

> 'I know you feel really strongly about this, and for the best of reasons, concern for your colleagues, so I'll formally log that the new risk profile is of great concern to you. But you need to come back and apologize when you've had five minutes to calm down. Or else come back tomorrow and I'll have to give you a written warning for verbal abuse. I can't allow you to talk to me like that, no matter what the circumstances or strength of feeling.'

When we talk about soft skills for supervisors, this is what we mean at the sharp end. It's also a great example of what has often been termed the 'supervisor squeeze', where they're in the situation of needing to 'make it so' without necessarily having the resources to do that easily or without impacting on risk levels.

One of the classic assertion books is *Games People Play* by Eric Berne. It has lots of examples of colleagues pretending to do one thing while doing another. For example, 'This is a wonderful empowerment opportunity for you . . .' translates as '. . . to do something I'd really rather not do myself because it's dirty, boring or scary'.

These are generic skills, but a workforce skilled at assertion is one where challenging unsafe behaviour and being challenged about unsafe behaviour is more likely to happen.

Case study

Here's an example of a company that took that approach to BBS and made it the centre of the strategy. It was called 'Middle Bubble Training' after transactional analysis (TA) theory, which says we can be in one of three states when interacting with others:

- parent;
- adult; or
- child.

The child state is only appropriate in a brainstorming session, but the parent state should also be avoided as much as possible. The style of an authoritarian parent shouldn't be confused with a directive leadership style, which is appropriate when employees are inexperienced or at risk, but often constitutes overuse of a top-down 'because I say so' mode. At its worst, an authoritarian style will engender a 'balancing' negative response, but even the more benign 'nurturing parent' style has two negative side effects.

First, if you assume you know best and are inevitably talking down to someone, it will inevitably hinder your listening. Second, it won't do the worker's empowerment any good.

The 'adult' state in this case is simply about assertion, active listening and giving good feedback, especially when that is negative. Helpfully, the model lends itself to a user-friendly triptych, as illustrated in the diagram below. It's very easy to think of things in threes: so, top bubble, middle bubble or bottom bubble? And the key principle is simple: the more often employees are in their middle bubble, the better.

Here's a true example of how user-friendly the model is. Twenty years ago, I still occasionally frequented places where people congregate to drink alcohol, look for sexual partners and listen to music. Late one night, a huge chap tapped me on the shoulder and said, 'You just spilled my pint'.

'I don't think so', I replied, sizing him up. 'Yes you did', he said, turning square on to me and leaning over intimidatingly. Trying to stay calm, I said, 'Look, I really haven't bumped into you or anyone else. You've got the wrong bloke'. Looking me in the eye from too close for comfort, he insisted, 'No, I've got the *right* bloke . . .' but then with a giggle '. . . but luckily for you I'm in my middle bubble and all's good! Ha . . . had you going there!' Thankfully, I recognized a trainee from a BBS course I'd run a few years before, a 6-foot 4-inch forklift truck driver with profound literacy issues.

Such generic skills facilitate the effective flow of analysis and communication, both of which are utterly central to creating a strong safety culture. They clearly fit under the 'nudge' banner, as they cost little but can have a big impact on behaviour. I mention this chap's literacy issues to stress how easy and appropriate it is to train everyone in interpersonal techniques that can sound complex and challenging in a textbook.

If we really want to create a culture where 'it's OK to be challenged and it's OK to challenge', we need to equip individuals with the skills to do that. As Reason suggests at the close of *The Human Contribution*, safety needs to be seen as a 'guerilla war'. We need to arm the troops as best we can.

Coaching

If you understand the *feedback fish*, you understand the basics of coaching. Imagine your 4-year-old has brought you a picture of a fish, but it's nothing better than an outline. Instinctively, you *wouldn't* exclaim, 'That's rubbish'. Instead, you'd say, 'Oh, that's fantastic . . . I'm so grateful you made the effort to draw me a fish. Thanks'. Then, because you want them to improve, you'll ask, 'I wonder, how could we make this picture even better? Let me think. How do fish see?' and the 4-year-old will shout, 'An eye! We need an eye'. Then, they'll add one in. In response to the question, 'Fish *swim*, don't they?' we'll get fins, and finally a fully formed fish.

It's the same with a safety conversation. Even though they know you know, so long as they say it first, they will have proved they knew it and will own it. Studies with electrodes monitoring brain function show it lighting up like a Christmas tree. Unless it's 'My God. Yes, brilliant . . . you're a genius', it doesn't do so when they say yes in agreement to a suggestion or recommendation from someone else. Basically, it's the same physiological response, just internalized for modesty!

'One in ten'

A builder of submarines won a BBS process of the year award by having a team of six tour the site and ask this question of a worker once a week. It's taken from educational psychology, where the counsellor tries to build on the answer 'I'd score myself 1 on a 1 to 10 scale as a student' by following up with the question 'How can we get that up to a 2?'

In coaching, when someone has said, for example, that they are an 8/10 at driving safely, the key is to ask why they aren't a 0, rather than why they aren't a 10. Then, when being told about all the good things they do, we can nod and smile, provide positive feedback and generally build rapport. So we can also say, 'My job as a safety coach seeking a step change is to get you from 8/10 to 9/10 and halve those unsafe behaviours'.

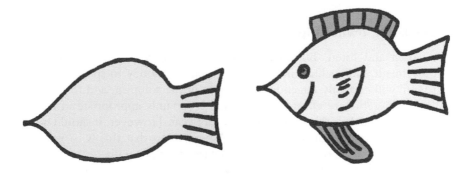

Figure 9.2 The two key principles of coaching illustrated by the 'Feedback Fish'

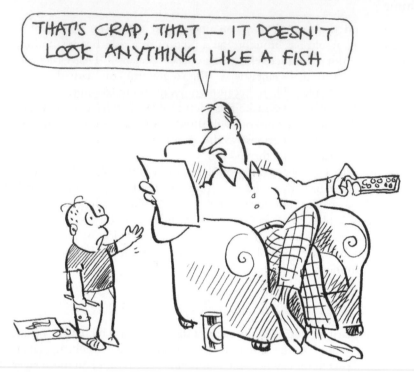

AS HIS COLLEAGUES COULD TESTIFY, BOB'S
COACHING STYLE LEFT A LOT TO BE DESIRED

Figure 9.3 A coaching opportunity missed . . .

We should have, by this point, minimized defensiveness and be primed to have a constructive discussion.

Engendering ownership

You coach and listen, but there needs to be clarity of thought between empowerment and egalitarianism. 'Here's a pot of money to spend, do so as you wish' will certainly engender ownership of the solution, add to the possibility of discretionary effort generally, and is certainly appropriate in certain circumstances, such as the choice of safety footwear. However, it should never tip into an abdication of responsibility. A perception that this is so will, for example, reduce the possibility of discretionary effort generally.

An excellent example of genuine ownership of a BBS process would be a shipbuilding company that offered a weekend for two in Amsterdam for a winning logo design. Many entries were received and the prize was won, but workers weren't impressed. 'Every day this ship is delayed costs them millions. What's a weekend for two in Amsterdam?' complained one employee, while others went further, alleging that the incentive was 'just a bribe, really'.

However, it was noticed that 11 entries were from children and, with a twelfth quickly 'commissioned' from the CEO's son, we had a calendar. This needed reprinting twice. With 2,000 workers on top of each other trying to get the platform finished, the job and the deadline were challenging, and the ship was only finally commissioned while being towed to its initial mooring, but there was not one single LTI.

Ownership comes primarily from choice and involvement. If you say it first, you own it, even if everyone knows you were led to the statement. So it's about the psychology of the leader member exchange and it's about perception. Management can't tell workers they have ownership; workers tell management. This is as much to do with one-to-one exchanges and soft skills as it is about delegation, roles and responsibilities.

Well-being, motivation and the undercover boss

If you've ever watched a version of the international TV show *Undercover Boss*, you'll have noticed that the boss always learns a lot and nearly always develops more respect and affection for their workers. It's a nice user-friendly validation of the techniques referred to earlier. However, it's also a variation on the old truism that it's impossible not to have at least some affection for a person whose story you know, and that links back to the holistic nature of safety, well-being and motivation.

Most programmes finish with a worker being promoted, and they always beam with smiles and announce they can't wait to tell their family. Often in these shows, the boss will go on to say, 'I'm just so thrilled to have someone like *you* working for me', and very often the employee will well up. More money is always really welcome after all, but that's a practical issue.

Being valued as a *person* gets you straight in the primeval reptilian brain. It means you're not likely to be pushed out of the cave anytime soon and are probably *safe*.

10 Systematic behavioural analysis

The simple principle of Five Whys analysis is that where a question 'why?' can be asked curiously, but in fact isn't, a learning opportunity is lost. Asking why *aggressively* isn't the same thing at all.

This 'curious why' technique really isn't difficult if you're at all 'mindful,' which is good news because, if you double the number of times it happens with your organization, you'll utterly transform your safety culture and standards.

That is if you have the commitment to do something with the analysis that comes back.

It's *five* whys because it's held that it takes a trail of five questions or less to get to the root cause of something.

It's a variation on the principle of six degrees of separation that suggests everyone is related to everyone else in six steps or fewer. Two or three whys will also quickly take you back up Reason's Swiss cheese model or the 'safety hierarchy'.

For example, Billy isn't wearing his safety specs. Why? Because they've misted up and he can't see what he's trying to do. Why? Because they are cheap and mist up easily, and the fact that the extractor fan is broken again isn't helping. The next why about the safety specs take us to the disclosure that the company bought cheap ones to save money, though it's now clearly proving a false economy. The solution is obvious, and we can also now explore the issue of the broken extractor fan.

The trick is to keep going, down as many avenues of inquiry as open up, until asking the question is pointless. We can keep going indefinitely of course, like a 4-year-old. However, 'Why did they want to save money?' isn't a question that really needs to be asked.

Nobody should be allowed to leave home without knowing about the power of the curious why question!

Applied ABC analysis

Let's plug that basic learning approach into something a bit more systemic.

Sometimes called 'applied behavioural analysis', this is the systematic application of our knowledge of ABC analysis, or how consequences and antecedents interact. As well as applying clever psychology, if it is carried out well, it also incorporates the safety hierarchy, brainstorming problem-solving, impact

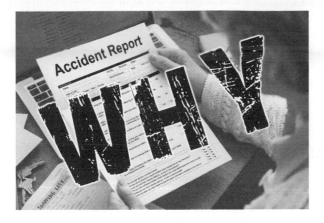

Figure 10.1 The curious why

Five Whys Analysis

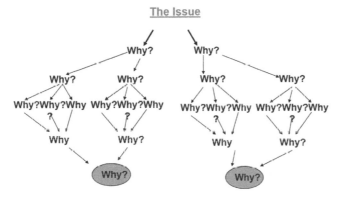

Figure 10.2 What a classic '5 whys' analysis might look like

matrixes and 'Five Whys' analysis to give as objective an answer as possible to the question: 'What happened? Why did it happen? What can we do to stop it happening in the future?'

Another name for this technique is 'temptation' analysis, and we can also use it entirely proactively with, for example, peripatetic workers assembled in a canteen, which directly addresses the conundrum of how you can apply behavioural safety to workers we cannot observe.

This isn't a 'nice to do' desirable on the essential/desirable list; it's a cast–iron essential and the very core of good BBS. For example, even when an organization simply cannot commit to an ongoing *process*, we can still undertake a behavioural safety *project* with this methodology as the basis of it. Training front-line workers or management in this then takes around one day:

- First, identify the suboptimal behaviour or situation you want to improve.
- Then brainstorm all the antecedents to the behaviour in question (i.e. the relevant triggers and contextual issues that preceded the behaviour).
- Then brainstorm all the consequences and potential outcomes.
- Finally, hold a mirror up to the situation by reversing it and doing the same for the same behaviour or situation when done *safely*.

We could use a template such as this:

Worked Example

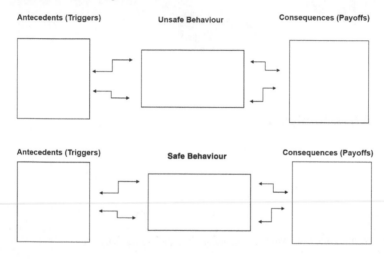

Figure 10.3 A systemic approach to ABC analysis

We could also seek to put the suggestions in a 2×2 matrix such as this:

Impact Matrix: (My very *favourite* lead measure).

	High	Low

E a s y	• 'Nudges' and other
	• clever, cost effective
	  design solutions
		• Posters and
		  inspirational talks

H a r d	• Effective but more
	  complex or expensive
	  solutions
		• Retrain everybody!

Figure 10.4 The 2 by 2 impact matrix

Essentially, this is the current situation systemically mapped out across a sheet as best we can. We ask the volunteers to undertake the following key step:

Score each of the consequences 0 to 3 based on:

- soon or delayed;
- certain or uncertain; and
- positive or negative.

For example, a *soon*, *certain* but *negative* combination would score a 2. This will quickly identify the real problem, where, for example, taking a shortcut through scaffolding and getting on with the job scores 3. It's *soon*, it's *certain* (rounding up regarding the small likelihood of injury causing disruption), and it's *positive* to the person involved. Falling scores just 1. It would, if that small likelihood came up, be *soon*, but it's unlikely and it's definitely negative!

This allows us to frame it as a football (soccer) score. And 3–1 is a solid win every time. It's also the *equivalence test* in action. What this scoring is saying is that, faced with the same situation, the average person will be tempted to cut the corner and 'crack on'. And we know that where there's temptation, it's just a head count from there.

Here's a real example.

We found a situation where workers who required new goggles would go to stores and climb a ladder to reach the boxes of goggles. These boxes were light, which is why they were on the top shelf. Frequently, it was noticed that the workers wouldn't be in quite the right place, so would take a firm grip and reach for the box. In doing so, they would violate the 'always keep your torso within the rungs' behavioural rule (i.e. no reaching) and score an 'unsafe' for anyone observing them with a check-sheet in their hands. It's a classic temptation to hold tight, reach and 'crack on'.

The golden rule when we're analysing ideas is that if the solution does not *directly address* this temptation, then it's not going in the 'high-impact' box, no matter what. Straight away, this helps with all sorts of biases and lazy thinking. Reason jokes that if you solved a problem successfully with a hammer last week, then next week everything is going to look like a nail!

The next step is to systemically work through the lists of antecedents for both negative and positive behaviours because, especially in the list of antecedents to the *positive* behaviour, the solution might be right there staring you in the face.

Here, the observation 'Operatives are not allowed to operate machine X without goggles' proved important.

It's important to restate that only solutions that *design out* the temptation to lean outside the ladder qualify for the high-impact column. Thus, constructing a mezzanine deck *does*, but retraining in the use of ladders *does not*. Moving frequently required items to the bottom of the storage rack *does*, but even extra supervisors with stun guns does not, as even in the latter case a small temptation remains.

The antecedent list might well suggest something further up the *safety hierarchy*, which is always a better place to be working. In this real-life example, someone asked, 'Why do you need goggles to operate machine X?' closely followed by, 'Why does machine X spit out swarf?' The answer was that it was an old machine that needed lots of servicing to keep it going and didn't come fitted with a screen. The next question asked was whether we could retrofit a lightweight Perspex screen, and indeed we could. Then someone asked, 'So, just how much does it cost to keep this lump of rusting junk running anyway?'

Although this final question is not unrelated to a proper long-term safety solution, it's not one to which I knew the answer.

This isn't an atypical example. In my experience, the project team will always be able to come up with a handful of 'high-impact, low-cost' (HILC) solutions. They will also be likely come up with a number of high-impact, high-cost solutions, but that's why directors of health and safety are well paid. The HILC solutions, however, are the very definition of '*investing* in safety', and should always be implemented as soon as possible. Otherwise, why are we bothering? More than that, workers who come up with analyses and solutions should be lauded in every available way possible, such as coverage in in-house magazines and praise in safety briefings.

Output:

We now have a number of key behaviours being undertaken safely far more often than they were previously.

We now have a body of even more highly motivated workers, who can, for example, be asked to volunteer for an ongoing observation-based BBS *process* with some degree of success.

We have some 'good news about safety' for a change that helps set a more positive 'yes we can' tone generally. We can cross-reference that 'it's OK to challenge and it's OK to be challenged' mantra and mindset that requires building. Indeed, clearly here we have all three key elements of a strong culture in action: empowerment, objective analysis and good leadership. Its ripple effects will be entirely positive.

Not bad for a day's training and a couple of hours a week for a month or so for a handful of workers.

Volunteers

It's worth addressing the concept of BBS volunteers. I agree that a volunteer is worth 10 pressed men, as the old saying goes, but a related point is worth mentioning.

It draws on Malcolm Gladwell's observation, in the book *The Tipping Point*, that everyone is equal, but some are more equal than others when it comes to change management. He calls these key change agents 'mavens'. Sometimes it is indeed worth taking someone of experience or charisma to one side and saying, 'You didn't volunteer yesterday and we were really hoping you would,' or even taking them to one side *before* the session and using flattery, bribes or just asking very nicely to prime them to surprise everyone with an early raised hand.

Often, we'll identify an individual with the intelligence, experience, charisma and credibility to be a perfect volunteer. Then we find that they did indeed volunteer several years ago but quit in exasperation. Getting someone like this to 'give it another go' and then show the commitment and support to ensure they don't regret it is BBS gold.

It must be stressed, however, that any bribes should be small and symbolic. Too big a bribe, and the individual may well agree but just go through the motions. That's not ideal.

What's great about getting someone to genuinely engage is that, as a bonus, as they undertake safety-related behaviours such as observation, challenging and analysis, their internal mental model shifts to one of being 'safe and proactive', and a virtuous circle is set up. The volunteer who, in the past, *usually* wore their PPE and who *usually* stuck to the prescribed walkway becomes someone who always does. The process of cognitive dissonance rears its head again. If this is someone with the ear of the canteen, then that's some proactive flattery or well-directed bribery.

Safety Differently and *Safety 1 and Safety 2*

It's worth at this point cross-referencing to the two important books in the subheading that have been published recently. These books are underpinned by three core principles:

- People are the solution, not the problem.
- Safety is the presence of positives, not the absence of negatives, with (drawing on positive psychology) a learning focus on what goes right.
- Safety is an ethical responsibility, not a beaurocratic necessity.

Safety 1, in essence, reflects a systems focus and learning from incidents. Proactive questions about 'What's inconvenient about doing this job safely?' are person-focused and proactive, but still addressing what might go wrong. *Safety* $1\frac{3}{4}$ perhaps? A *Safety 2* question would be 'What do I need to do to help you do this job safely?' or 'What happens when things are safe and efficient?'

A simple practical example of applying the '2' principle would be that safety briefings/toolbox talks and the like must contain a minimum of 20% dialogue, thus ensuring that the workforce involved interact and contribute, and cannot simply sit mute and uninvolved then sign the form that's passed around to confirm 'attendance and understanding'.

Another key principle is the acceptance that most companies have too many rules, and that many of them are simply not followed by the workforce, even if they know about them! This is illustrated perfectly by one presenter, who shall remain nameless for the purposes of discretion, who tells the story of the site tour with a CEO. The CEO expressed himself thrilled to see the workers following the safe systems of work and method statements, even though 'they are clearly not finding it easy and are making a big effort' (i.e. it must be as their 'hearts and minds' had been won!). The guide pointed out that they were following them because the CEO was touring, and struggling with them as they were implementing them to the letter for the very first time.

Indeed, to an extent, the '2' view is that talking about 'hearts and minds' is actually offensive, as it suggests that people are getting hurt because they don't care enough about their own safety. Worse, in some cases, this 'safety' mantra of 'hearts and minds' can become like a religion, where no dissent is allowed and where people questioning any underlying principles can be seen as heretical. For example, anyone questioning 'zero harm' can be accused of 'accepting that people will get hurt', with this possibly becoming a self-fulfilling prophecy. In short, 'your lack of faith is condemning someone to get hurt'. Who wants to be guilty of that?

Again, a *Safety 2* view would take a more rational view and point out that glorying in a low LTI rate and zero paper cuts when the building is about to blow up makes no sense, and that effort and resource must be targeted proportionally at the most important issues. (Getting the balance right between process and personal safety was discussed under the section on Heinrich's principle above.) Certainly, no one rational would disagree that effective proportionality is more important than repeating mantras blindly.

What's certain is that the books, by Dekker and Hollnagel respectively, have generated much debate in the world of safety. Indeed, some people have started asking, 'Are you 1 or 2?' in the tone of a McCarthy witch-hunt, with only one acceptable answer. A more nuanced and appropriate answer is, '2 of course, whenever possible and appropriate'.

To summarize this short overview, I'd argue that the theme of this book, as with these two books, builds explicitly on the Just Culture work of James Reason (and of course Dekker's own earlier work). The books *Safety Differently* and *Safety 1 and 2* both encourage an interactive and proactive approach that fit comfortably with the analysis and facilitation approach championed here.

Dekker, S. (2015) *Safety Differently*. CRC Press.
Hollnagel, E. (2014) *Safety 1 and Safety 2*. Ashgate.

11 Lead and behavioural measurement

When running a research project in Manchester, we tried really hard to develop behavioural measurement as a science, and were commissioned by the UK Health and Safety Executive to train a team of its inspectors in the techniques. I still haven't come across anything as advanced, so I'll share those techniques here, of course, but before doing so it's worth making some predictions and observations:

- Lead measures often sound valid, but in truth are vague and can suffer a disconnection from reality on the shop floor.
- Behavioural lead measures are the best lead measures as they enjoy the strongest direct correlation with risk and harm, or the least disconnect.
- Collecting good-quality data isn't especially difficult. The techniques, I hope, will sound sensible and achievable.
- Good-quality behavioural data can also be used for goal-setting sessions, as well as tracking and resource directing.

However:

- Really good-quality behavioural data is as rare as hen's teeth.
- This doesn't stop many an organization entering poor-quality data into very expensive computer programs that generate lovely graphs and charts.

As the US Civil War general's envoy said, pre-empting 'garbage in, garbage out' comments about computer analysis, 'The general accepts that the intelligence is unreliable and of poor quality, but keep supplying it please as he needs it for planning purposes'.

Lead measures

Where does behavioural data fit within the lead measure framework?

According to the extensive and free-to-use Campbell Institute website (www.thecampbellinstitute.org/research), lead measures should be *proactive, predictable* and *preventative*. Other adjectives often required of them, it says, include actionable, achievable, explainable, meaningful, timely, transparent, useful and valid. I'm not sure whether such a list scores most highly for thorough and useful, overlapping or intimidating.

Regardless, three broad sets can be identified:

- *Operations* such as risk assessment, compliance, corrective action closeout, change management and training.
- *Systems* would include permit to work, surveys, disciplinary issues and hazard analysis.
- *Behaviour*, our primary focus here, including leadership, front-line engagement, 'walk-and-talk' and other 'visible' methodologies.

As ever, it's not the existence of such processes, but the quality, that counts. I'd like to pick an operations and systems example to illustrate the observation that, despite some very sexy-looking graphics, they actually tell us nothing of much use.

In an improving culture, hazard-spotting metrics increase. It's well documented that first aid and even injury rates often increase as the culture improves. A less obvious example would be a training metric such as 'percentage of employees trained compared to percentage of employees we intended to train'.

We can see from the example above that we have halved the number we missed last year, and can congratulate ourselves on our achievement. It's a fun course, delivered with passion by entertaining trainers, so the happy sheets look great too. We have several impressive-looking charts to wave at the C-suite and visiting auditors.

However, several questions remain:

- Was the training based on an astute gap analysis of need, just considered useful by one individual, or something that used up the budget to ensure next year's isn't cut? Or was it just something to wave at a regulator?
- What percentage of the at-risk population are we talking about? All of them or just some? Are contractors included?

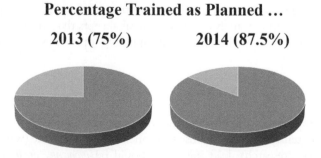

Percentage Trained as Planned …

2013 (75%)   **2014 (87.5%)**

Figure 11.1 Percentage trained as planned

- Were there any language or comprehension issues? For example, 'I am new here, the trainer was nice and so I gave him a good score even though I didn't understand much'.
- Were the messages clear and sticky so that 'what to do' is remembered several months later?
- Was 'Why we need you to do this more/less' covered in enough depth for the delegate to demonstrate some 'operational dexterity', should the situation not be clear-cut?
- Were the new behaviours requested practised to the extent that individuals left feeling confident enough to attempt them in action when given the chance? Highly skilled and engaging trainers role-playing at the front, so that delegates can watch and say, 'Yes, I see what you mean' isn't the same thing as actually *practising* it.
- Were the behaviours requested followed up on-site so that opportunities to use them draw negative feedback if missed and positive feedback if taken?
- Was the training followed up by line managers and coaches so that early attempts to use new skills could be discussed and any support required could be actioned?
- Did we follow up to ensure that the behaviours happening more/less often deliver something unambiguously positive for the organization? Or are they just something different, or even worse, because of an unintended consequence?

Even this isn't an exhaustive list, but it does make the point that simply asking an employee 'Have you been trained?' and 'How was the course?' and getting the responses 'Yes' and 'Great, actually' doesn't necessarily prove much.

Many a pie chart based on 'lead measure' data looks convincing and face-valid. The simple question that underpins all good science must be rigorously asked and researched. Is this *causation* we are looking at, or merely *correlation*? And if causation is claimed, then how can we *prove* it's the case?

Surveys

Surveys are a good way to proactively find out what's going on.

My experience, however, is that the tick-box survey suffers from two huge problems. First, the person filling it in cares about it somewhat less than the people who wrote it, and there's the issue of who will analyse the data. This means a certain amount of random ticking.

Second, a typical respondent will not believe for one minute that the survey is anonymous, and therefore may well second-guess the answers they think they ought to best supply. This is especially true of electronic surveys.

Combined, this usually results in huge amounts of error variance, meaning that a score of 50, plus or minus 5, needs to increase to a score of 80, plus or minus 5, before we can be *certain* that things have genuinely improved.

Face-to-face culture surveys are much better, as the respondents, who are usually in groups, can be assured personally that the pollster doesn't want to know their names, there are no right or wrong answers, and the purpose is just to find out what they *think*, why they think that, and to hear some examples. This provides really rich data and gives a really clear warning to the researcher if the first answers are 'best foot forward', or even an excellent opportunity to knee-jerk 'diss' the company in any way.

Here is a typical example of our own culture survey, with the management scores above and workforce scores below. In *both* cases, the groups seemed motivated and honest, so it illustrates the need for a proper sampling methodology that covers all elements of the organization!

To paraphrase, management is saying:

'We like to think we're not too bad actually, and are particularly strong in the areas of analysis and communication.'

While the workforce is saying:

'b*&^%cks'.

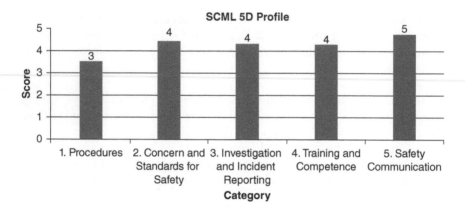

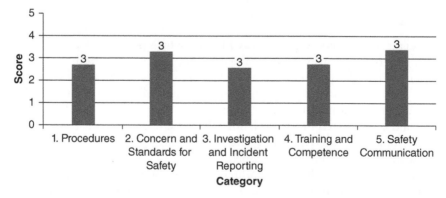

Figure 11.2 Client data showing typical scores and a classic workforce v. management inconsistency

Unless the discrepancy is so great as to show that management is utterly deluded, it matters not that scores diverge. What's important is *what we learn from them*. Indeed, exactly why management and workers disagree is merely one of a number of hugely fruitful learning opportunities.

The symbolism of conducting a survey has an impact too under the heading 'What gets measured gets done' because it tells the workforce what we're interested in. A caveat to add to that is that how well we measure it and how well it appears we are measuring it impacts on that. If it is a valid measure and if it is also a face-valid measure, then it's well worth doing.

Here's an interesting case study demonstrating the power of what gets measured gets done. Examples above have illustrated the principle that 'we get what we demonstrate we want' and taking the trouble to measure it demonstrates that want. This example, from an Italian manufacturing plant, adds an amusing refinement to the famous 'what gets measured gets done' truism.

Unless we don't do anything with the findings, in which case unintended consequences kick in, and we'd have been better off doing nothing!

Effectively applying the learning from such data will impact significantly on front-line risk, and is therefore 'behavioural safety'.

This final section is about out-and-out 'behavioural measurement' as it's typically understood. I hope you'll find that this section is as at least as in-depth a coverage of behavioural measurement as anything available in the literature.

Behavioural measures

What's especially good about front-line behavioural measures is their point-to-point correspondence with outcome. Here are two examples from clients of ours.

ITALIAN MANUFACTURING PLANT

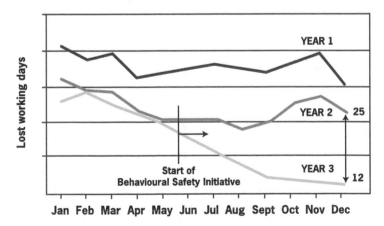

Figure 11.3 What's *about* to be measured also gets done

Case study 1: manufacturer

The first chart shows the mean scores for a variety of categories: housekeeping, PPE, worker/machine interface, etc., which caused the vast majority of incidents for this client. There were a variety of easy wins to be had here. For example, the pedestrian door that would remain locked most of the day unless you found the keyholder and asked them to open it.

You can tell from the incident rate that this was a very rough-and-ready industry with a lot of challenges, but management commitment was high because of a fatality. The point I'd like to make here is that the ratio of scores going up and accidents coming down is very closely correlated, so there's no need for any cross-referencing and caveats, as with the training pie charts above.

Case study 2: chemical manufacturer

This second example is even simpler, as it involves just one simple behaviour and just one very cheap solution. That said, this had been going on for years, and their parent company was extremely well known.

At this plant, the vast majority of days lost were to burns and dermatological issues because there were lots of instances when workers would need to manually handle containers of caustic soda, which is all this site manufactured. Sometimes they'd not wear gloves when they did this, and sometimes the containers leaked.

We found that only one size of glove was provided because it was cheaper than supplying a variety of sizes, and no one had ever complained. People with

BEHAVIOURAL SCORES AND LTI RATE

Note improvement ratios are almost identical (23.5 to 8.2 and 10.3 to 2.5)

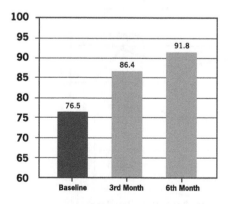 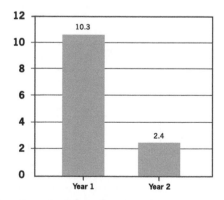

Figure 11.4 Client data showing how accidents decrease when behavioural scores increase

big hands couldn't get the gloves on and people with small hands found the fingers flopped about in an inconvenient way.

The solution to provide three sizes of glove was cheap, and its impact on days lost (their favoured lagging measure of safety) was dramatic.

Again, it's the correlation between the two sets of data that I want to consider. As unsafe acts relating to key behaviours reduced, so did harm. In both cases, understanding why unsafe acts occurred led to simple, cost-effective changes that enabled an improvement in performance.

We just need to focus a solution-based, not blame-based, approach directly on the appropriate behaviours. The workforce will always understand and be able to explain the underlying causes and what needs to be done to rectify the situation. It just needs a little listening. Or we could send all workers on a fire-walking course and say, 'If you can do this, you can do anything, so be safe'.

Accurate behavioural measurement

Here's an example of 'if we can measure it, we can manage it'. It's from a utility company that had thousands of walkways across dozens of sites. Many were degraded and hazardous, but efforts to improve matters were piecemeal. Often contractors couldn't be bothered to quote for small jobs, and the paperwork required was offputting. In this case, we were provided with a team of BBS assessors who toured the whole site scoring each 40 yards of walkway against agreed standards, who came back with thousands of data points. The feedback session to senior management proved both interesting and productive.

SAFETY PERFORMANCE
(BEHAVIOURAL MEASURES AND WORKING DAYS LOST)

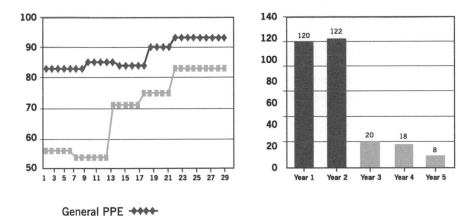

General PPE ◆◆◆◆
Job specific PPE ▪▪▪▪

Figure 11.5 Another client's data showing the inverse relationship between behaviour and harm

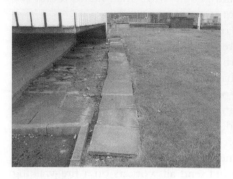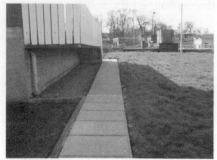

Figure 11.6 What gets measured gets done

It must be noted that the benefit of 'what gets measured gets done' doesn't always require accurate measurement, though it's important that it is considered reasonably accurate measurement, or else it will lack even face validity and the workforce will just ignore it.

However, many practitioners such as BST describe the classic BBS model as:

- Identify the key behaviours.
- Measure them.
- Feed back the results.
- Remove the barriers.

Clearly, if we base our approach on this model, then accurate measurement is key, as it is for Geller's 'DOIT' approach, which stresses 'I' is for intervene and 'T' is for 'test that the intervention worked'.

Specifically, accurate measurement allows:

- benchmarking against other organizations/other parts of the organization/ other shifts;
- meaningful goal-setting sessions to describe accurately 'where we are now' and define 'where we want to be'; and
- the impact of training, design solutions, and other initiatives and processes to be objectively assessed.

All things considered, it's clear that *accurate* measurement of front-line behaviours is a good thing and better than no measurement. My experience, however, is that achieving it in the medium- to long-term is far more difficult than most people realize.

I'll try to justify that sweeping statement.

Imagine two observers tasked to go out with a check-sheet asking to look for behaviours relating to PPE, housekeeping, the interaction of people and machines, and movement about site because we know from analysing the data and talking to employees that if we can crack these items, we have covered 80% of all lost time incidents. Consider that they are both sensible, experienced, diligent and motivated, though this can be something of an assumption in places where ownership of or the perceived credibility of a BBS approach is poor.

Observers A and B walk around the site scoring what they see, diligently, and put their observations into a spreadsheet, where the week's data is collated and turned into a sexy-looking pie chart or bar graph. Here is a list of the things that can put error variance into the behavioural data system because even diligent, experienced people may well see two different things. What I think is common sense and what you think is common sense may differ wildly.

Classic problems with checklists that generate error variance:

1 There are vague item definitions

The item definitions are vague – 'Make sure people are using the stairs safely' or 'Make sure people are wearing overalls correctly', for example.

If the question 'What exactly do you mean by that?' can be asked, then the definition is too vague. For example, with overalls, you may need to say that:

- they are done-up to the neck;
- they have sleeves rolled down and outside of gauntlet gloves;
- they have trousers outside of boots;
- nips are allowed up to 2 cm, but no tears that could snag or let in splashes; and
- they must not be overly impregnated with oily waste.

2 Photographs are required

Where it's virtually impossible to define 'overly', as above, we need borderline photographs to illustrate where acceptable falls. Importantly, these should not be good and bad examples that mean 'picky' people will use the good photographs as the standard to work from, as 'anything worse than that fails', while more laissez-faire types will gravitate towards the bad example on the basis that 'anything better than that is OK'.

3 Generic rules are needed

Two observers could watch a forklift truck driver working hard for two minutes and see dozens of individual movements, many of which might be borderline in terms of being acceptable or unacceptable. Was that too quick a turn? Was that engagement a bit too bumpy? One observer scoring these harshly and one scoring leniently could come up with wildly diverging scores. A generic rule, while it would reduce sensitivity, would greatly enhance consistency.

For example:

> Watch the driver for two minutes. If they transgress any of the following key points, fail them; if not, pass them. Then go and watch five other drivers and come back with six marks in total.

A similar rule might be applied to any rapid-fire frequent behaviour, such as the use of hand-operated tools or manual work on a production line.

4 Maps for housekeeping items

Maps are always useful for telling observers how many housekeeping marks to give in a specific area. For example, make clear that an area (a room or a designated part of a big room) gets one mark and a section gets another to ensure that one person doesn't score every pile of boxes and every extinguisher, and another person just the room.

Walkways can, for example, be scored as 'circa 30 m long', so a standard 25 m walkway gets one mark and a 100 m walkway three or four marks, depending on the location of user-friendly 'border points' such as doors, side paths or drainpipes.

5 People forget to score the safes

It might be that even though all data is collated and turned into an overall percentage, one observer, for example, watches 20 scaffolders access a build and scores it as '8 safe and 2 unsafe'. However, we know that unsafe actions leap out at us in these circumstances, so a second observer, only 'seeing' these two miscreants taking a shortcut access to the site, scores it 2 unsafe.

6 A lack of technical knowledge

A subset of this error-inducing issue is where an observer is watching something technical. Whether a worker has a hard hat on or not is easy to score, as is whether employees are holding the handrail or not. But items relating to the use of specialist tools or lifting operations on a drill floor are harder, especially if, for example, you're a cook.

We've often found that observers don't feel comfortable 'judging' colleagues when they're a bit uncertain, and simply decline to give a mark either way. What's needed here is some cross-function peer-to-peer coaching in what to look for.

It was during one such session that one of my favourite observer training stories occurred. Being shown around a kitchen, a driller was shown an emergency stop button. He took the cook up to the drill floor and, paraphrasing the 'That's not a knife; this is a knife' quote in the film *Crocodile*

Dundee, said 'What you showed me isn't an emergency response button; *that's* an emergency response button' pointing out something rather larger and more user-friendly.

7 Poor sampling

The sampling 'catch-22' can often apply. We know how to sample accurately, as around the world exit polls accurately predict an election result minutes after a poll has closed.

The trouble is that, like water always taking the easiest route down a hill, observers will, left to their own devices, get into a user-friendly pattern, and we'll get scores that will, for example, tell how safe the site is just after lunch on a Tuesday when it's nice and quiet and safe, but most convenient for taking an observation. We most need to take observations when it's usually the least convenient time to do so, as people are stretched and busy, and that's when gaps in the system announce themselves.

This simply needs planning effort and management commitment. An example of this would be the client that used random number tables to ensure that operatives could never predict when and where an observer would appear. There was much amusement when one observer 'drew' 10 a.m. and 11 a.m. on Monday morning.

Accuracy and consistency checks

In the Manchester project, we tried very hard to design out the faults described above by, for example, feeling it right to sacrifice a little sensitivity for the consistency that robust 'generic rules' brought. In order to check how well we were doing with this, we designed the 'accuracy and consistency' methodology. The UK HSE was impressed enough to ask us to train a team of officers in the techniques.

What we found was that achieving 'really good data' was indeed possible, but almost no organization had the appetite for it long enough to collect high-quality comparison data over any sort of meaningful amount of time.

We found that sometimes inconsistencies evened themselves out so that two different observers could come back with a similar percentage. However, if this didn't also reflect a similar *number* of scores, then that agreement would be highly unlikely to be repeated. We found that if a simple cross-check with agreement for both the percentage score *and* number of observations made were both above a coefficient 0.9 meant then the data was solid. If either of these fell below 0.8, we felt that was too much error variance.

The basic A&C methodology was for two or more observers to go out and score the same site without any sort of communication. By communication, we meant eye contact, nods, pointing, winks, thumbs up and other 'what do you think?' non-verbal communications.

Here's a real-life example:

Accuracy and Consistency Data

	A		B	
	Safe	Unsafe	Safe	Unsafe
1. Lifting operations / use of tools	4	0	0	0
2. Workbench tidiness	10	1	1	10
3. Fork lift truck operations	2	2	24	2
4. Walkways	23	48	1	17
5. Movement around site	31	2	0	2
6. Walkways and emergency equipment	15	5	19	1
	59% (143)		58.5% (77)	

Figure 11.7 Accuracy and consistency data

As you can see, the similarity in percentage is fine, scoring a coefficient of 0.99 (58.5 divided by 59). However, it's highly unlikely to be repeated as the coefficient score for the *number* of marks given is only 0.5 (77 divided by 143). The method from here is simply to 'eyeball' the data – honestly a technical term meaning taking an objective overview – identify where the discrepancies are, discuss why they occurred, agree a remedy, then, of course, rerun the A&C check to make sure the remedy actually works.

The problems we found in order:

- *Lifting operations*: Observer A, an FLT driver, simply didn't feel comfortable judging this task. (Solution: technical training required.)
- *Workbench tidiness*: Observer A passed anything half-decent. Observer B, on the other hand, failed anything with any problems. (Solution: a borderline photograph was required.)
- *Forklift operations*: Observer A was giddy from trying to score each individual movement, but Observer B will have been using a generic rule.
- *Walkways*: Observer A scored each pile of boxes and each trip hazard – finding lots of 'safe bits' and lots of reasons to fail an area, but scoring them all. However, Observer B was working to a map with a generic rule of 'if there's anything wrong, fail it'.
- *Movement about site*: Observer A simply failed to notice the many staff moving about safely.
- *Emergency equipment*: In this example, we found that there were maps, generic rules and example photographs in use, but the definitions and

photographs weren't as pinpoint as they could be. You can see that this resulted in one observer scoring this 95% safe and the other only 75%.

Crucially, this amount of variation isn't much use regarding a goal-setting session, which starts with the observation, 'Overall, we're at 80%; we hope to halve that and get to 90% in the next three months'.

Three observations:

1   I don't think we've ever had a client that could point to A&C scores that passed muster for more than three or four months.
2   This didn't stop many from turning observation data into sexy-looking pie and bar charts and using these in meetings with no caveats. Many also used the data in goal-setting sessions over a period of years.
3   This also didn't stop some investing in very expensive computer tracking programs. We even had one we provided ourselves. It was reasonably priced by comparison to others, but even so we took an executive decision to stop selling it.

Behavioural benchmarking

Being able to practise what we preach and to objectively and accurately compare different clients/different factories or regions, or to track the effectiveness of processes and initiatives over time, is extremely useful. Scoring the six most important items on a site and benchmarking them against established norms always provides a simple graph, which is very interesting to clients.

There are contact details on the back of this book somewhere if you'd like our help with that, of course, but I'd hope you now have everything you need to generate accurate data on that in house.

Goal-setting and feedback sessions

If the data collected is accurate enough to be credible then, as well as feedback charts and the like, a goal-setting session is possible. Ideally, this will be run by the workforce themselves, with colleagues assembled in a canteen to debate and agree a hard but realistic goal. Following this, charts can be updated weekly to track progress towards this goal.

A well-attended and motivated session such as this can be a hugely important event in the BBS process. This is especially so when someone astutely observes, 'We can get from X to Y in two months, no problem, but we'll need Z to achieve it'. This occurred most spectacularly in my experience when baseline scores for bypassing interlock gates, and some other machine interface issues, were presented at a factory in Manchester, and the workforce were genuinely stunned at how bad things had got. After an excellent discussion with some astute observations, a target much higher than we were hoping for was agreed, and it was hit the following week. Job done.

Things that can go wrong:

- The chart isn't updated promptly every Monday morning as promised, but can stay unchanged for weeks on end. The unintended consequence is that this is now a well-placed and colourful reminder for all the lukewarm commitment to the process by either management or the volunteers, who perhaps merely fancied a couple of days away in a hotel for a training course.
- The session is led by management, and the attendees agree with anything suggested but don't actively participate in any meaningful way. Thus, an opportunity to engage the workforce in the process is lost.
- The session is run in a coaching style and by peers too, but clumsily, so that a response to a 'surely we can do better than that?' prompt is something such as, 'Look, why don't we just cut to the chase and you tell us what target you want us to agree to. Then we can all clear off and get back to work'.

Very explicitly, I'm suggesting some basic training in the generic interpersonal skills described above for all involved in such a process. Again, covering the underpinning psychology helps with that all-important operational dexterity we want as obstacles arise in the process.

Cultural measurement

Earlier in the book, I mentioned my own simple model of safety culture, and objectively scoring the behaviours associated with that ongoing process of *culture creation* is actually quite easy. It's like a proper culture survey, but more rough and ready. We simply need to wander the site asking people a handful of key questions. For example, we know that praise is a key part of the coaching element of transformational leadership ('catch a person doing something right'). So we might simply ask a cross section of people which of the following five anchors most often applies.

Praise for safe behaviours

5   At least once a day (and *far* more than you criticize).
4   Several times a week (and more than you criticize).
3   Maybe once a week (on balance with criticism).
2   Once in a while (less than you criticize).
1   Never.

Similarly, when looking at the 'asking why' aspect of *learning mindfully*, we might ask people to pick a response from the following. In this case, anchoring only *every other* number, which some people who develop Likert scales prefer, as it makes deciding on a response more user-friendly.

Use of 'curious why'

5   It is the default around here, and I agree that when something has gone wrong, it is analysis first and foremost.

4

3   Often used, but often there will be an assumption of lack of effort.

2

1   Management say it's a 'no–blame culture', '. . . but . . . they really like to know who they aren't blaming'.

Please forgive the use of humour at the end of each point, but in truth each check-sheet should be tailored and designed to discriminate people within *your* organization. Where your baseline is will dictate which way the anchors should be skewed, with 'always' perhaps ludicrously optimistic from the off. Or it could be that 'never' is unduly pessimistic.

For example, how often does your supervisor lead by example? For a currently *weak* culture:

5   Nearly always.

4

3   Usually.

2

1   Sometimes.

Or, how often does your supervisor lead by example? For a *strong* culture:

5   Always.

4

3   Nearly always.

2

1   Usually.

Other suggested questions

•   To what extent does the organization proactively ask, 'Anything slow, uncomfortable or inconvenient about doing this task safely?'

From a leadership perspective:

•   When discussing an issue that needs addressing, to what extent does the organization adopt a coaching technique (i.e. using a questioning technique to draw out the individual's knowledge and maximize the chance of 'discovered learning')?
•   To what extent does the leadership lead by example?
•   To what extent does management convey a clear and convincing desire for a strong safety culture?

It's not the person, it's the environment, so please note that these scores are local–environment–sensitive. A rating of 'nearly always' in a *weak* culture will almost certainly reflect a high level of *individual* effort and integrity. Conversely, a rating of 'usually' in a *strong* culture would nearly always indicate an individual who has yet to 'get with the programme'.

This sort of follow–up assessment is the very core of any culture improvement programme, which is BBS. Everything mentioned above is a behaviour that impacts on how much risk will occur. We've identified a need to improve and senior management has bought in. We've rolled out good-quality training to all, and everyone left the room promising never to fail to lead by example. How systematically and thoroughly we follow this up, praising when we find people behaving as promised, and coaching (and/or punishing) those that aren't, will cover 80% of the efficacy in the medium- to long-term.

Setting up workforce behavioural analysis teams is my very favourite approach to cultural improvement, and these teams look just fantastic in front of visiting insurance companies and clients. They're not as important as this basic follow–up work, though.

A bold prediction

Halve the gap between where you are now for just the top seven leadership behaviours described above, and I guarantee an utterly transformed culture. Most importantly, I predict this improvement will be confirmed if you cross-check by measuring the top six most risky front-line behaviours.

To be crystal clear: If you start with the behaviours, any decent behavioural *analysis* approach will far more often than not take you straight to the issues on this list, because 9 times out of 10 unsafe workforce behaviours are a symptom of a weak culture, and not a cause in themselves.

Clearly, I'm advocating a holistic BBS approach where you do both.

Conclusion

This brings us to the end of my attempt at an overview of BBS in its many varieties. The key points are:

- Since everything impacts on behaviour, then *everything is BBS*. Every conversation, the words spoken and the way they are spoken contributes to the safety culture, and therefore to the likelihood of whether an unsafe act occurs or not. So does everything we do and the way that we do it. As indeed does what we think and the way we think about things.
- Taking this holistic approach allows for a more joined-up and realistic set of methodologies.
- This allows us to address the very notion of zero harm and the risks of an 'LTI-free' obsession, and address driver safety, home safety and process safety, as well as well-being and mental health issues.

- The word 'behaviour' sets us off on the wrong foot from the start, and should be avoided if possible.
- Unless we objectively understand why an unsafe behaviour has occurred, we cannot effectively invest in improvement. Training in basic ergonomics and human error, in Just Culture and in such things as the law of unintended consequences, must be the first thing we do.
- Observations and measurement, if used at all, simply tell us how well we're doing this. It should be observations as part of a learning approach, not learning as part of an observation approach.
- That simple-sounding sentence actually refers to a profound mindset shift with fundamental implications for BBS methodologies.
- There's a lot of time, effort and money invested in BBS that is BS. From sexy-looking pie charts spat out from ludicrously expensive computer programs based on poor-quality data, through to fire-walking courses that end with the entirely person-focused statement that 'If you can do that, you can do anything – so off you go and be safe'.

And finally:

- This holistic approach to behavioural enhancement – a total culture perspective – minimizes the possibility of us blowing the place up on the same day as we award ourselves a prize for being LTI-free.

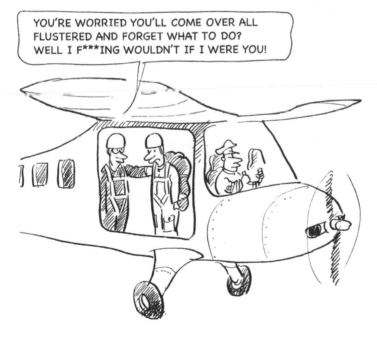

Figure 11.8 Sound advice delivered directly and unambiguously

That just leaves it to me to thank you for your attention. I'd really like to wish you good luck, and the Irish blessing that the 'winds of good fortune be ever at your back'. But that rather contradicts everything that's been said above.

'Now look, you'll probably just be getting the luck you deserve' is no way to finish a book, is it?

Suggested reading

I have tried to summarize and, more importantly, *synthesize* much of the key thinking in the following excellent and influential works with direct reference to BBS or the behavioural change methodologies suggested in this work. In the spirit of this book, please feel free to both validate that claim for yourself and to point out where I've gone wrong!

Ajzen, I. (1991) 'The theory of planned behaviour'. *Organizational Behaviour and Human Decision Processes*, 50(2).

Alter, A. (2013) *Drunk Tank Pink*. Oneworld.

Blanchard, K. and Johnson, S. (1982) *The One Minute Manager*. William Morrow.

Bryson, B. (1998) *Notes from a Big Country*. Black Swan.

Clarke, S. (2013) 'A meta-analytic review of transformational and transaction leadership styles as antecedents of safety behaviors'. *Journal of Occupational and Organizational Psychology*, 86(1).

Conklin, T. (2012) *Pre-Accident Investigations*. Ashgate.

Cooper, M.D. (2009) *Behavioral Safety: A Framework for Success*. BSMS

Daniels, A. and Agnew, J. (2010) *Safe by Accident?* Performance Management Publications.

Dekker, S. (2006) *The Field Guide to Understanding Human Error*. Ashgate.

Dekker, S. (2007) *Just Culture*. Ashgate.

Deming, W.E. (1986) *Out of the Crisis*. MIT Press.

Geller, E.S. (2000) *The Psychology of Safety Handbook*. Lewis Publishing.

Geller, E.S. (2015) 'Behavior based approaches to occupational safety'. In *The Wiley Handbook of Occupational Safety and Workplace Health*. Wiley Blackwell.

Goldstein, N.J., Martin. S.J. and Cialdini, R.B. (2007) *Yes! 50 Secrets of Persuasion*. Profile Books.

Heinrich, H.W. (1959) *Industrial Accident Prevention: A Scientific Approach* (4th edn). McGraw-Hill. (Note that in 1969, a Frank Bird, working for the Insurance Company of America, collated similar figures but published no formal papers.)

Hellier, E., Wright, D.B., Edworthy, J. and Newstead, S. (1999) 'On the stability of the arousal strength of warning signal words'. *Applied Cognitive Psychology*, 3.

Hellier, E., Wright, D.B., Edworthy, J. and Newstead, S. (2004) 'Linguistic and location effects in compliance with pesticide warning labels for amateur and professional users'. *Human Factors*, 46.

Hersey, P. and Blanchard, K.H. (1969) 'Life cycle theory of leadership'. *Training and Development Journal*, 23(5).

Hopkins, A. (2008) *Failure to Learn*. CCH Australia.

Hopkins, A. (2012) *Disastrous Decisions*. CCH Australia.

Kahneman, D. (2011) *Thinking Fast and Slow*. Farrar, Straus & Giroux.

Kotter, J. (1996) *Leading Change*. Harvard Business School Press.

Krause, T. (2005) *Leading with Safety*. Wiley.

Marsh, T. (2014) *Talking Safety*. Gower.

McSween, T. (1995) *The Values Based Safety Process: Improving Your Safety Culture with a Behavioral Approach*. Van Nostrand Reinhold.

Parker, D., Lawrie, M. and Hudson P.T.W. (2006) 'A framework for understanding the development of organizational safety culture'. *Safety Science*, 44(6).

Pavlov, I.P. (1927) *Conditioned Reflexes: An Investigation of the Physiological Activity of the Cerebral Cortex*. Oxford University Press.

Pink, D. (2005) *A Whole New Mind*. Riverhead Books.

Reason, J. (1997) *Managing the Risks of Organizational Accidents*. Ashgate.

Reason, J. (2008) *The Human Contribution*. Ashgate.

Ross, L. (1977) 'The intuitive psychologist and his shortcomings: distortions in the attribution process'. In L. Berkowitz, *Advances in Experimental Social Psychology 10*. Academic Press.

Schneider, B. (1987) 'The people make the place'. *Personnel Psychology*, 40.

Sinek, S. (2013) *Leaders Eat Last*. Penguin.

Skinner, B.F. (1953) *Science and Human Behavior*. Macmillan.

Syed, M. (2010) *Bounce*. Fourth Estate.

Syed, M. (2015) *Black Box Thinking*. John Murray.

Taleb, N. (2007) *The Black Swan*. Random House.

Thaler, R.H. and Sunstein, C.R. (2009) *Nudge*. Penguin.

Vroom, V. (1992) *Management and Motivation*. Penguin.

Interesting reading

Books that have one or all of the themes: objectivity, learning, data, efficacy, psychology. (Or, if you found this book at all interesting and/or useful, I promise you'll find these interesting and/or useful!)

Berne, E. (1964) *Games People Play*. Penguin.

Carter, P. (2007) *Don't Tell Mum I Work on the Rigs: She Thinks I'm a Piano Player in a Whore House*. Da Capo Press.

Gladwell, M. (2000) *The Tipping Point*. Abacus.

Gladwell, M. (2005) *Blink*. Penguin.

Gladwell, M. (2013) *David and Goliath*. Allen Lane.

Hallinan, J.T. (2009) *Why We Make Mistakes*. Broadway Books.

Levitt, S. and Dunbar, S. (2005) *Freakonomics*. Penguin.

Levitt, S. and Dunbar, S. (2009) *Superfreakonomics*. Penguin.

McFarlin, B. (2004) *Drop the Pink Elephant*. Capstone.

McRaney, D. (2012) *You Are Not So Smart*. One World.

Index